About the author

Jennifer Worth trained as a nurse at the Royal Berkshire Hospital, Reading, and was later ward sister at the Elizabeth Garrett Anderson Hospital in London, then the Marie Curie Hospital, also in London. Music had always been her passion, and in 1973 she left nursing in order to study music intensively, teaching piano and singing for about 25 years. Jennifer died in May 2011 after a short illness, leaving her husband Philip, two daughters and three grandchildren. Her books have all been bestsellers and have been translated into more than twenty languages.

Suzannah Worth is the elder of Jennifer's two daughters. Following Jennifer's death, she and her father devoted their time to keeping Jennifer's work and memory alive. Suzannah trained in special needs education, has taught clarinet and worked in libraries. She plays clarinet in the Hemel Symphony Orchestra and sings in a local choir. In her spare time she enjoys baking, pottering in the garden, cycling, swimming and yoga. Suzannah lives in Hemel Hempstead and has two daughters and one Godson. Inspired by her mother, Suzannah is now writing her first book.

Toffee Apples and Quail Feathers

The best of *Call the Midwife*

Jennifer Worth

Compiled and with a foreword by Suzannah Worth

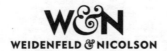

WEIDENFELD & NICOLSON

This edition first published in Great Britain in 2022 by Weidenfeld & Nicolson
This paperback edition published in 2023 by Weidenfeld & Nicolson,
an imprint of The Orion Publishing Group Ltd
Carmelite House, 50 Victoria Embankment
London EC4Y ODZ

An Hachette UK Company

3 5 7 9 10 8 6 4 2

A CIP catalogue record for this book is
available from the British Library.

ISBN (Mass Market Paperback) 978 1 3996 0188 7
ISBN (eBook) 978 1 3996 0189 4
ISBN (Audio) 978 1 3996 0995 1

Typeset by Input Data Services Ltd, Somerset
Printed in Great Britain by Clays Ltd, Elcograf S.p.A.

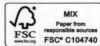

MIX
Paper from
responsible sources
FSC
www.fsc.org   FSC® C104740

www.weidenfeldandnicolson.co.uk
www.orionbooks.co.uk

IN MEMORY OF MY PARENTS
Jennifer Louise Worth
1935–2011
and
Philip Lloyd Worth
1933–2019

May Flights of Angels Sing Thee to Thy Rest

This book is dedicated to my wonderful sister Juliette
and my two beautiful daughters, Lydia and Eleanor

Contents

FOREWORD

In which we discover the story behind
Toffee Apples and Quail Feathers

Whether you are already a fan of Jennifer Worth and her writing or are new to it: hello and welcome. First of all, a little bit about my mother Jennifer, her life, her work and her writing. You will find some interesting and useful background information, which hopefully will fill in a few gaps and answer a few questions you may have.

How did it all begin? Well, in 1998, quite by chance, my mother came across an article in the *Midwives Journal*, exploring the representation of midwives in literature; or rather the lack of it. The article finished with a challenge: 'Perhaps there is a midwife out there somewhere who can do for midwifery what James Herriot did for vets.' My mother was the midwife who rose to that challenge. She sat herself down at the table in the dining room and started writing, with a pot of strong coffee and some dark chocolate to keep her going.

Once she started writing she couldn't stop; she wrote on scrap paper with her trusty fountain pen (she hated biros), correcting mistakes as she went with little bits of white sticky paper, because she was too impatient to wait for correction fluid to dry. She wrote furiously for two or three hours at a time, and then, if the weather was nice, would go out for a bike ride, for a breath of fresh air and to plan her next chapter. That's when she did her best thinking and she kept a little notebook and a pencil in her saddlebag to jot down ideas.

Sometimes she took herself off to her flat in Brighton (Hove, actually) to do her writing. Here, instead of a bike ride, she would go for a swim in the sea to do her thinking and planning. She had another notebook and pencil in her swimming bag so she could jot down any ideas that came to her while she was doing battle with the waves.

The job of typing her manuscripts fell to her adoring husband, my adorable father Philip Worth: one-time clerk for various small-time law firms; latterly a teacher of Classics, Economics and Law; and, in his retirement, an artist. He had little choice in the matter really because my mother had a fear of computers and wouldn't touch one with a bargepole; nor would she pay someone to do the typing for her.

My father acquired a computer, and, with a rudimentary grasp of how it worked, he made a start. It's fair to say it didn't come naturally to him, but it was a labour of love, and despite numerous mistakes he laboured on. He knew how to type (albeit slowly) and how to save a document. He could use a few of the functions but not all. Someone had told him how to highlight everything by pressing ctrl+A, which he found useful. Unfortunately, no one thought to tell him the purpose of ctrl+Z (undo) which, as time would tell, would have been much more useful.

I clearly remember him spending hours typing up a particularly long chapter ('The Captain's Daughter' from *Farewell to the East End*), which, for some reason, he highlighted when he got to the end. He then pressed another key at random and, in the process, wiped the whole chapter before he'd managed to save it. All would have been well if he had known the purpose of ctrl+Z but he didn't, so after swearing furiously at the computer, a brisk walk to clear his head and a stiff whisky, he set to and typed the whole thing again, bless him.

After three years of writing, typing, editing and proof-reading, which fell to me (my mother liked to keep it in the family), *Call the Midwife* was ready for publication. But that was not the end of it, and she kept on writing until two more books were published: *Shadows of the Workhouse* and *Farewell to the East End*, which collectively form *The Midwife Trilogy*. All three books became international bestsellers, and inspired a hit BBC television series by the same name. But that was still not the end of the story and she kept on writing, with a fourth book in mind. In 2010, *In the Midst of Life* was published, which also became a bestseller.

But then the unthinkable happened: early in 2011, my mother, who had been having trouble swallowing for some weeks, was diagnosed with cancer of the oesophagus. By the time of her diagnosis the tumour was so large she could no longer swallow anything, not even fluids. She had a stent inserted to open up the oesophagus, so she could get some nourishment down her, but that was it; she refused surgery to remove the tumour, preferring to let nature take its course. We were all in shock, my father in complete denial; my mother, who a few months previously had been swimming in the sea and riding her bike, was going to die. She came home and we cared for her until she died just two months after her diagnosis.

A few months after her death, with Episode One of the first TV series soon to be transmitted, my father and I were asked if we would like to give a talk at the local library, where I was working at the time. The talk was a great success, word spread and more and more requests started coming in, so we decided to take *Call the Midwife* on the road. Together with our good friend Andrew, who acted as presenter, we gave talks at literature festivals, in libraries all over Hertfordshire, to WI groups and at fundraising events. It was a marvellous time for both of us; it was a tribute to my mother, keeping both her work and her memory alive.

We always gave a reading at our talks, our favourite and undoubtedly the most popular being 'Sister Monica Joan gets stuck in the bath' from *Farewell to the East End*, with Fred the boiler man in the starring role. My father, who had a great sense of humour and could do a brilliant Cockney accent, played the part of Fred. His timing was impeccable and he knew just when to drop the punchline: '*Well, I reckon as 'ow I must be the only bloke in England wot's seen a nun stark naked.*' As you can imagine, our audiences burst out laughing, and it took several moments before we could resume the reading.

Life changed significantly for both of us when, in 2016, I moved back into the family home to take care of my father, who was getting more and more frail. Life fell into a familiar routine and one evening we were sitting in his study, he with his brandy and me with a white wine and tonic spritzer, chatting about this and that. For some reason the subject of middle names came up. He confessed to feeling more than just a little aggrieved that he hadn't been given one at birth. His older brother and younger sister had middle names, but he did not; the middle child with no middle name. We decided there and then to do something about it, and so he selected Lloyd (in honour of his father) to be his middle name. There is no official record of this anywhere, which is why I have chosen to remember him in this book as Philip Lloyd Worth. So here he is immortalised; I can hear him chuckling now.

Despite his frailty, we continued our talks; he struggled into the venues, leaning heavily on his Zimmer frame, but, as soon as we sat down, he would come alive and entertain our audiences with his easy charm and delightful sense of humour.

In 2019, eight years after my mother's death, at the age of eighty-five, my father fell and broke his hip. He had surgery, but, because he was so frail, he 'failed to thrive', to use the proper medical term. Three weeks after his fall, my sweet, kind and gentle father died in hospital, with my sister and my two daughters in constant attendance. It was a peaceful, dignified death, which is all any of us can hope for. It was a privilege to live with and care for him in the last years of his life, and I still miss him dreadfully.

In January 2020, the unimaginable happened: there were reports of a deadly virus, which initially seemed a long way from home but within weeks had swept across the world, and in March 2020 we were all thrown into something called 'lockdown'. The government watchwords were: *Stay Home. Protect the NHS. Save Lives.* Social contact outside of households was forbidden; only essential shopping was permitted and, thankfully, 'daily exercise' for one hour per day. Thank goodness for daily exercise, because that's what kept me going. When my mother died, I inherited her bike; when we were thrown into lockdown, I got the bike out, pumped up the tyres, oiled the chain, worked out a few pleasant routes through the countryside, and off I went. Daily exercise sorted.

They say history repeats itself. As I was peddling along with nothing but birdsong all around, I found myself using the time to think, just as my mother had done all those years ago. How would my parents have reacted to the pandemic if they were still alive? They would probably have had little awareness of it, as neither of them watched the news or read the papers. My mother may well have carried on regardless, because that's the kind of person she was. My father would not have had a problem staying home, because he hardly ever went out anyway, but he would certainly have missed our talks and visits from all his friends.

Another day and another ride; as I was cycling along, thinking about this and that, it suddenly dawned on me that 2021 would be the tenth anniversary of my mother's death. There must be something we can do, I thought to myself, to mark the occasion somehow; to celebrate her life and her writing. And then I remembered, tucked away in the back of a drawer, a folder of unpublished material.

When my mother died, the job of sorting out all her paper-work fell to me, mainly because I am local and my poor father was too overcome with grief to know where or how to begin. I made a start and it soon became clear it was going to be a monumental task. My mother kept every piece of written material that she thought might be of value or importance at some point in the future. Not only were there dozens of folders of all her handwritten and typed manuscripts, there were also publishers' drafts of all of them. There were books, magazines, journal articles and newspaper cuttings, all of which she used when doing research for her books. I filled a small cupboard and several drawers with her manuscripts, and rationalised the books, articles and cuttings.

I found a folder full of handwritten letters, which, on close inspection, I realised were from people who had read her books and wanted to share their own stories with her. Evidently these letters were very important, as she'd replied to every one of them, dating each letter when her reply was sent. I didn't feel it was my place to get rid of this collection and so I tucked it away in the back of another drawer. As it turned out, it was a jolly good thing I didn't get rid of these letters because a few years later they formed the basis of the book *Letters to the Midwife*.

It took quite some time to sort and organise everything, and it wasn't until several months after her death that I came across two more folders: one a mysterious handwritten manuscript with no title; and the other a typed manuscript simply labelled 'Fifth Book'. A fifth book? Needless to say I was curious, and so I made myself a cup of tea and sat down to read this so-called fifth book. I thought it was brilliant. There it was, the makings of another book by Jennifer Worth. This is too good to be true, I thought, but what to do with it? With no immediate answer to that question, I tucked both folders away in the back of yet another drawer (fortunately we have a lot of drawers) and put it to the back of my mind . . . until my lockdown bike ride, that is.

I hurried home from my ride as quickly as possible to start the search for both folders. With so many drawers to go through, it took a little while, but eventually I found what I was looking for. It appeared to be a collection of stories featuring Fred the boiler man. I checked the folder of handwritten material against the folder labelled 'Fifth Book', and sure enough they were one and the same. With mounting excitement, I reread all the material. Some of the stories were fully formed and typed up, some were not yet typed. Some were incomplete and some were just ideas, but there was enough material for half a book. If these stories were carefully edited, and combined with a selection of favourite stories from the trilogy, I thought, we would have the perfect book to celebrate my mother's life, her work and her writing. But was I up to it? With the tenth anniversary of her death approaching, I decided it was time to shine the spotlight on her writing once again, and so I rose to the challenge. I sat myself down at my desk in the sitting room and started the tricky but rewarding job of editing, with a cup of camomile tea and a piece of flapjack to keep me going.

With the editing complete, I needed to come up with a title, and what better than two of Fred's little earners? To complement the new material, I have selected additional stories from the trilogy, featuring two of my favourite characters: Chummy and Sister Monica Joan. So, welcome to Fred's world, to his odd jobs and little earners; to fireworks, to toffee apples and quail feathers. Welcome to the world of pigs and manure and allotments. My hope is that this book will give you as much pleasure as I have had in bringing it together.

Suzannah Worth

PART I
FRED

In which we meet Fred

In this chapter, taken from *Call the Midwife,* we are introduced to Fred for the first time and some of his 'little earners'. My mother paints a wonderful picture of Fred, which my father took great pleasure in describing to our audiences when we gave our talks. In the same chapter we are introduced very briefly to Mrs B the cook and also to Chummy. The year is 1957, when my mother joined the community of Nonnatus House to complete part two of her midwifery training.

Chapter One

FRED

A convent is essentially a female establishment. However, of necessity, the male of the species cannot be excluded entirely. Fred was the boiler man and odd-jobber of Nonnatus House. He was typical of the Cockney of his day and age: stunted growth; short bowed legs; powerful hairy arms; pugnacious; obstinate; resourceful – all these attributes were combined with endless chat and irrepressible good humour. His most striking characteristic was a spectacular squint. One eye was permanently directed north-east, whilst the other roved in a south-westerly direction. If you add to this the single yellow tooth jutting from his upper jaw, which he generally held over his lower lip and sucked, you would not say he was a beautiful specimen of manhood. However, so delightful was his optimism, good humour and artless self-confidence that the Sisters held him in great affection, and leaned on him heavily for all practical matters. Sister Julienne had a particularly strong line in helpless feminine appeal: 'Oh Fred, the window in the upper bathroom won't close. I've tried and tried, but it's no use. Do you think . . . ? If you can find time, that is . . . ?'

Of course Fred could find time. For Sister Julienne, he would have found time to move the Albert Docks. Sister Julienne was deeply grateful, and praised his skill and expertise. The fact that the window in the upstairs bathroom was fixed permanently closed from that time onwards was no inconvenience, and not mentioned by anyone.

The only person who did not respond with delight to Fred's particular brand of Cockney charm was Mrs B, who was a Cockney herself, had seen it all before, and was not impressed. Mrs B was Queen of the Kitchen. She worked from 8 a.m. to 2 p.m. each day and produced superb food for us. She was an expert in steak and kidney pies, thick stews, savoury mince, toad-in-the-hole, treacle puddings, jam roly-poly, macaroni puddings and so on, as well as baking the best bread and cakes you could find anywhere. She was a large lady with a formidable frontage, and a particular glare as she growled, 'Nah then, don' chew mess up my kitchen.' As the kitchen was the meeting point for all staff when we came in, often tired and hungry, this remark was frequently heard. We girls were very docile and respectful, especially as we had learned from experience that flattery usually resulted in a tart or a wedge of cake straight from the oven.

Fred, however, was not so easily tamed. For one thing, the orientation of his eyes being what it was, he genuinely could not see the mess he was making; for another, Fred was not going to kowtow to anyone. He would grin at Mrs B wickedly, suck his tooth, slap her ample bottom and chuckle, 'Come off it, old girl.' Mrs B's glare would turn into a shout. 'You ge' out of my kitchen, you ugly mug, and stay ou'.' Unfortunately Fred couldn't stay out, and she knew it. The coke stove was in the kitchen, and he was responsible for stoking it, raking it out, opening and shutting the flues, and generally keeping it in good order. As Mrs B did much of her cooking, and all of her baking, on that stove, she knew that she was dependent on him, so a strained truce prevailed between them. Only occasionally, about twice a week, a shouting match erupted. I noticed with interest that during these altercations neither of them swore; no doubt this was out of respect for the nuns. Had they been in any other environment, I felt sure the air would have been blue with obscenities.

Fred's duties were morning and evening for boiler stoking and extra time by arrangement for odd jobs. He came in six days a week for the boiler, and the job suited him very well. It was a steady job, but it also allowed him plenty of time to pursue the other activities he had built up over the years.

Fred lived with his unmarried daughter Dolly in the lower two rooms of a small house backing on to the docks. He had been called up during the war but, due to his eyesight, had been unable to enter the armed services. He was therefore consigned to the Pioneer Corps, where, if Fred is to be believed, he spent six years serving King and Country by cleaning out latrines.

Compassionate leave was granted to him in 1942, when his wife and three of their six children were killed by a direct hit. He was able to spend a little time with his three living children, who were shocked and traumatised, in a hostel in North London before they were evacuated to Somerset, and he was ordered back to the latrines.

After the war, he took two cheap rooms and brought up the remains of his family single-handed. It was never easy for him to find a regular job because his eyesight was erratic, and because he would not commit himself to being away from home for long hours – he knew that his children needed him. So he had developed a wide range of money-making activities, some of which were legal.

Fred's best line, with the highest profit margin, had been fireworks. His unit of the Pioneer Corps had been attached to the Royal Engineers (REs) in North Africa for a time. Explosives had been in daily use. Anyone, however humble, working with the REs is bound to learn something about explosives and Fred had picked up enough to give him confidence to embark on fireworks manufacture in the kitchen of his little house after the war.

'S'easy. You just need a load of the right kind of fertiliser, an' a touch of this an' mix it wiv a bi' of that an' bingo, you've got yer bang.'

Chummy said, wide-eyed with apprehension: 'But isn't it frightfully dangerous, actually, Fred?'

'Nah, nah, not if you knows what you is a-doin', like what I does. Sold like nobody's business, they did, all over Poplar. Everyone was wantin' 'em. I could've made a fortune if they'd left me alone, the bleeders, beggin' yer pardon, miss.'

'Who? What happened?'

'Rozzers, police, got 'old of some of me fireworks an' tested 'em, an' sez they was dangerous, an' I was endangering 'uman life. I asks you – I asks you! Would I do anyfing like that, now? Would I?' He looked up from his position on the floor and spread out his ash-covered hands in innocent appeal.

'Of course not, Fred,' we all chorused. 'What happened?'

'Well, they charged me, din't they, but the magistrate, he lets me off wiv a fine, like, because I 'ad three kids. He was a good bloke, he was, the magistrate, but he says I would go to prison if I does it again, kids or no kids. So I never done it no more.'

We had seen Fred in the market selling onions, but did not know that he grew them. Having the ground floor of a small house gave him a small garden, which was given over to onions. He had tried potatoes – 'no money in spuds' – but onions proved to be a moneymaker. He also kept chickens and sold the eggs, and the birds as well. He wouldn't sell to a butcher – 'I'm not 'aving no one take 'alf the profits' – but sold directly to the market. He wouldn't take a stall either – 'I'm not paying no bleedin' rent to the council' – and laid a blanket on the floor in any space available, selling his onions, eggs and chickens from there.

Chickens led to quails, which he supplied to West End res-taurants. Quails are delicate birds, requiring warmth, so he kept them in the house. Being small, they do not need much space, so he bred and reared them in boxes, which he kept under the bed. He slaughtered and plucked them in the kitchen.

His most recent economic adventure had been in toffee apples, and very successful it was, too. Dolly made the toffee mixture in the little kitchen, while Fred purchased crates of cheap apples from Covent Garden. All that was needed was a stick to put the apple on, dip it in the toffee, and in no time at all rows of toffee apples were lined up on the draining board. Fred couldn't imagine why he hadn't thought of it before. It was a winner. Nearly a 100 per cent profit margin and assured sales with the large number of children around. He foresaw a rosy future with unlimited sales and profits.

A week or two later, it was clear that something had gone wrong from the silence of the small figure crouched down by the stove, manipulating the flue. No cheerful greeting, no chat, no tuneless whistle – just a heavy silence. He wouldn't even respond to our questions.

Eventually Chummy left the table and went over to him.

'Come on, Fred. What's up? Perhaps we can help. And even if we can't, you will feel better if you tell us.' She touched his shoulder with her huge hand.

Fred turned and looked up. His north-east eye drooped, and a little moisture glinted in the south-west. His voice was husky as he spoke.

'Fevvers. Quail's fevvers. Tha's wha's up. Someone complained fevvers was stuck to me toffee apples. So, food safety boffins come an' examined 'em an' said fevvers an' bits of fevvers was stuck to all me toffee apples, an' I was endangerin' public 'ealth.'

Apparently the health inspector had asked at once to see where the toffee apples were made, and when shown the kitchen, in which the quails were regularly slaughtered and plucked, had immediately ordered that both occupations be discontinued, on pain of prosecution. So great was the disaster to Fred's economy that it seemed nothing could be said to comfort him. Chummy was so kind, and assured him that something else would turn up, something better, but he was not reassured, and it was a glum breakfast that morning. He had lost face, and it hurt.

But Fred's triumph was yet to come.

In which we meet the young Fred

These next five chapters are the first of the new, previously unpublished material, where my mother introduces us to the young Fred. We learn a little about his early life and the colourful characters he meets along the way. Crucially, we discover how his 'little earners' came into being. The stories take us from the turn of the century to 1932 or thereabouts. Had my mother lived long enough to finish the fifth book, I have no doubt she would have filled the gap between 1932 and 1957 with more stories of Fred, his odd jobs and little earners. We can only imagine what we are missing.

Chapter Two

THE YOUNG FRED

Fred was an only child, born at the turn of the twentieth century – his father had died shortly before he was born and his mother had never married again. 'I'm too busy working for courting,' she had said, laughing. They were always laughing in their one small room, never heated in the winter, when the ice covered the window pane. What little money she managed to earn during those lean years was spent on the rent, a few clothes to keep them decent, and food, the best of which she gave to her son.

School had been a bit of a nightmare, because he looked so odd and children can be so cruel. He was undersized, underweight and bandy-legged, but his most spectacular feature, however, was his squint. How he ever managed to get around was more than anyone could conjecture – he could see northeast in one direction and south-west in the other, but not in the middle. In order to look straight ahead he had to turn his head sideways.

He found that being the classroom joker helped, and this was a habit adopted in his first decade that stayed with him for life and became part of his character.

When he was just fourteen years old, his mother died from overwork and malnutrition – Fred thought his world had come to an end. He had an aunt and uncle, but they had seven kids in two rooms, and no work. They couldn't take another one to house and feed, so Fred had to make shift for himself.

Getting work was hard for everyone, and for the young Fred it was well-nigh impossible. His odd appearance put people off – they thought he was being saucy or perhaps shifty when he wouldn't look at them. But he *couldn't* look at them. He had to turn sideways to look at a person, which was decidedly off-putting. A lot of people laughed at him, which hurt him deeply, and there was no one to go home to; no mother to give him a hug and laugh the hurt away, and say, 'It's what's inside that matters, not the outside.' He couldn't get a regular job of any sort, so he took to odd-jobbing, and the habit stayed with him for life.

It was while he was sweeping up fish heads, bones and scales at Billingsgate Fish Market that he met Frank, a boy a little older than him, who was everything Fred had ever wanted to be. Frank was tall, good-looking and strong. He was confident and self-assured. He was a fish coster in his own right, not just a boy working for a man. Although only sixteen, Frank had been independent for two years and had made enough money to support his sister Peggy, who was only twelve and still at school.

To the scrawny, insecure Fred, Frank was invariably kind and friendly. He never laughed at him, never tormented him about his appearance, for which Fred, accustomed to being bullied by big boys, was deeply grateful.

Frank gave him a lot of work, and suggested jobs that would never have occurred to Fred, such as hiring a burner and selling roasted chestnuts to crowds in the winter, or in summer selling fizzy lemonade, which he showed Fred how to make from water, sugar, bicarbonate of soda and a shred of lemon. It was good fun and Fred began to enjoy the company of other people. He gained in confidence and stopped trying to hide his face.

The friendship between the two boys became something

of a fixture. Frank, clearly flattered by Fred's admiration, also enjoyed his quick wit, his unexpected idiosyncrasies and his very individual style of humour. Fred in turn blossomed in his friend's company, and his eccentricity, of which he was quite unaware, came to the fore as he became less inhibited.

He slept at night in a common lodging house, which was very rough and dangerous for a young boy, and one day Frank, who knew the score, said to him, 'Look 'ere, mate, you wants to get out of there or one day somefing nasty'll 'appen. There's an attic room going cheap in our place. You could take it – you're earning enough money to pay the rent. Why not?' So Fred took it and that was when he first met Frank's sister Peggy. She was the first girl he had got to know really well, and he liked her. She was kind and pretty and he developed quite a crush on her, but never dared speak of it. Their friendship gave Fred the security he needed and also the confidence to talk to a girl.

Fred had two regular odd jobs, if an odd job could be described as regular! His favourite was the job of boiler man at Nonnatus House, a community of nuns based in Poplar, with a busy nursing and midwifery practice attached. The job involved little more than raking out and stoking the boiler, but 'boiler man' sounded like a proper job and Fred was very proud of the title. Nonnatus House was essentially a community of women, so Fred had plenty of opportunity to talk to the fairer sex, but there was little hope of meeting the right kind of girl within the hallowed walls of a convent. There were the nuns, of course, who were kind and more than happy to talk to Fred, but nuns were nuns, after all, sworn to a life of poverty, chastity and obedience! The young nurses were another matter: pretty and chatty but incredibly busy, and they barely gave Fred a glance as they rushed about their business, let alone found the time to talk to him!

His other regular odd job involved the cleaning out of soap

scum from the pipes and drains of the local wash house, before the next day's washing came in. The first laundrette to be opened in this country was in 1949, in Queensway, London. Before that, laundry, if it was not done at home, could be done at washing stations within the wash house. The Poplar wash house was opened in 1852, in the East India Dock Road, and that's where Fred met young Maisie, who worked there.

Maisie was a cheerful soul and they enjoyed each other's company. They shared a dislike of the lady who supervised the wash house, who spoke with an affected posh accent, and Fred and Maisie liked to mimic her when they thought she wasn't listening. She was prim and proper and had a very superior attitude, especially towards Fred, who she thought was an impudent fellow.

One evening, Fred was called in by the supervisor lady to clear a blockage in one of the pipes. Fred was delighted – he had recently acquired a new set of rods, of which he was very proud, and he was keen to try them out. After much pushing and prodding, it still wouldn't clear so Maisie came over to see what was going on.

'Somefing's stuck,' he muttered. 'Wot if I goes up the other end and pushes the rod down, instead of up? That should clear it.' He told Maisie to stay where she was to keep an eye on the end of the pipe. The supervisor lady was hovering nearby to keep an eye on Maisie.

With every ounce of his puny strength, and much grunting and puffing, Fred continued to push and prod until suddenly, with tremendous force, something shot out of the end of the pipe and hit the supervisor lady clean in the face. It was an old sock, very wet and slimy, and stinking as only something that has been stuck in a pipe for several days can stink.

What followed the sock was a gush of smelly, slimy water, which soaked everyone's feet. Fred and Maisie roared with laughter; the supervisor lady, who was wearing a smart new pair of shoes, was furious. 'Oh, how disgusting!' she cried. 'Clear up this mess at once.'

'Oh, how disgusting!' Fred and Maisie mimicked, and laughed even harder.

'Maisie Sullivan, I have never been so insulted in all my life,' the supervisor lady said coldly. 'Take notice to leave at once. You are sacked.'

'Sacked?' whispered Maisie.

'From this moment. Get your shawl and leave, and you, Fred, never darken these doors again.' And with that she stormed out and slammed the door.

Fred and Maisie weren't laughing quite so much now – in fact, Maisie was pretty close to tears. Fred, who had a kind heart, hated to see Maisie so upset, so he gave her a quick hug.

'Well, I might have lost me job today, but I reckon as how I've found meself a boyfriend,' said Maisie cheekily.

'What, really! You mean me? You wants me to be your boy-friend?' said the incredulous Fred.

'Not 'alf,' said Maisie. 'I likes you.'

Chapter Three

MAISIE

Maisie was a sparky young girl, with high colouring, bright eyes and a mass of frizzy hair that she was always trying to tame, but with no success. She was only fifteen and had been working in the wash house for nearly two years. The money she earned was a pittance, but the few shillings she took home each week were essential to her mother's household economy. Younger brothers and sisters had to be fed and Father was out of work again. Losing her job was a serious matter.

'Fred, I've lost me job! What's me mum gonna say?'

'Don't you worry, Maisie, there's lots of things what you can do – no, what *we* can do to earn money. I know of loads of ways, and me mate Frank knows of loads more. We'll go and see him.'

Frank and his sister Peggy lived in the same house as Fred. Their parents had both died when they were tiny and they had both spent their early years in the workhouse. When Frank was eleven he had been apprenticed to a costermonger from whom he'd learned the trade. Frank was quick to learn, and by the age of fourteen he decided that he was not going to waste his young life being a coster's boy. He would be a coster in his own right, buying and selling for his own profit.

Spurred on by the determination to get his sister out of the workhouse, he worked from five in the morning till ten at night to save the money to redeem her. It had been a long, hard struggle but, by the time she was twelve, he had saved enough money, and rented a room that they could call home. They lived together all their lives.*

Fred and Maisie climbed the stairs to Frank's room. It was dark and so Maisie took Fred's hand. His heart soared; he had never held a girl's hand before.

'So you really are me girlfriend then?' he whispered. She didn't reply but squeezed his hand harder.

'Give us a kiss then,' he said, to test the water. She giggled and kissed his cheek.

'You wouldn't if it wasn't dark. Girls don't think I looks the part – they've told me so.'

'Well, you looks the part all right for me,' she said confidently.

Fred was overjoyed and gave her a smacker on the lips, an interesting experience for Maisie, no doubt.

Fred looked quite different when they entered the room, and Frank and Peggy noticed it at once. Gone was the apologetic hangdog expression, and replacing it was an ecstatic lopsided grin. Proudly, he announced, 'This is Maisie. She's me girlfriend.'

Together, they explained the predicament of Maisie losing her job; Fred making much of the story, pulling faces, and mimicking 'Oh, how disgusting' and 'never darken these doors again'. Frank and Peggy were helpless with laughter.

Maisie was laughing, but not quite so much. The sober reality was beginning to weigh on her.

'But I've lost me job,' she sniffed, 'and I've gotta go home soon and tell me mum, and what's she going to say? She'll half kill me, she will, when she hears.'

Fred stopped arsing about and looked down at his forlorn little girlfriend. He took both her hands in his and then had to turn his head sideways in order to look her in the eyes.

---

* For the full story of Frank and Peggy see *Shadows of the Workhouse*.

'Then don't tell 'er,' he said seriously. 'You don't 'ave to. If you goes out each morning at the same time and gives 'er your money at the end of the week, she'll never know.'

Maisie looked only partly reassured. 'But if I don't get me wages, how can I give 'er the money?'

'There's loads o' ways of earning an honest penny – nothing dishonest, like. I'm just saying there's loads o' ways we can earn a living, which could be a lot more fun than slaving away in the wash house for ten hours a day.'

He gave her one of his special grins. 'That's wha' we've come to see Frank for. He's an ideas man.'

'Well, I knows me way round and I've got a few ideas,' said Frank modestly. He was a bit older than the others and his nonchalant, streetwise attitude impressed them all.

'Well, now, let me see.' He paused and his audience sat forward eagerly. 'There's the ordinary sort of jobs, like winda-cleaning, painting 'n' decorating, office cleaning and the likes, but I suppose you want somefing a bit more lively, like?' Fred and Maisie nodded.

'Well, I suppose you could try guided tours of the East End like, or tours of the docks, or of Billingsgate Market. People love that sort of thing. You could hire a boat and do trips down the Thames.'

'That sounds real good,' interrupted Maisie.

'It is, I've seen them – ladies and gents out for the day. But you'd need capital to hire a boat, so maybe somefing else to start. You could try dog walking – everyone has dogs and no one wants to walk them. People would pay you to do it. Then of course there's collecting dog turd for the tanners and horse droppings for the gardeners.'

Maisie wrinkled her nose and Fred rolled his eyes. 'No, thanks,' they said in unison.

Frank stopped his discourse. 'Hang on a minute mate, do that again.'

'Do what again?'

'That thing you just done with yer eyes.'

'What thing I just done wiv me eyes?' said Fred, rolling his eyes. Maisie and Peggy screamed with laughter.

'That thing! Honestly mate, yer face is yer fortune – you could earn any amount of money in the music halls. Can you dance?'

Fred shook his head.

'I can,' said Maisie eagerly.

'Can you sing?'

'I reckon so.'

'So can I,' chorused Maisie.

'Can you play anything?'

'A mouth organ,' said Fred.

'A penny whistle,' said Maisie.

'There you go, you've got yerselves an act,' said Frank triumphantly. 'All you need is a stage.'

Fred jumped up and took Maisie for a little twirl around the room. 'We'll be in the music halls,' he chanted happily.

'Hang on a minute,' said Frank cautiously. 'You won't get in the Halls straight away – you need practice. What you needs to do is work up yer act and try it out on the people queuing to get their tickets. You could collect money in a hat after. Go on, I'm tellin' yer mate, it's a winner, straight up.'

Fred and Maisie worked up an act of sorts, with which they entertained the people queuing for their tickets, more for their enthusiasm than any skill or artistry. All went well for a few weeks until the theatre manager banned them; apparently there were complaints from the real stars of the show that they were being outshone!

Chapter Four

LITTLE EARNERS

Fred and Maisie made good money entertaining the queues, and were disappointed when it came to an end; now they would have to find another little earner. They decided they made a good team, and so would give one or two of Frank's other suggestions a go, but which to choose? Maisie liked the sound of boat trips and so they made a plan.

'Wot we needs is to see 'ow it's done,' said Fred. 'It's no good going into somefing like this wivout a bit of preparation.' Maise nodded eagerly.

With a little money saved from entertaining the queues, they bought two tickets for one of the many boat trips that regularly go up and down the Thames.

Maisie decided to sit near the guide, the better to hear the commentary. Fred decided to go up to the front of the boat, near the wheelhouse, the better to observe the skipper.

They set off, passing famous landmarks along the way; all the while the guide offering informative commentary. Maisie was impressed, but thought there was a bit too much history for her liking and not enough humour. With a bit of practice and a few cheeky Cockney jokes thrown in, Maisie reckoned she could give it a go.

Fred stood to the right of the wheelhouse and watched the skipper closely. It looked easy enough; all you had to do to go straight was hold the wheel with both hands near the top – at ten to two, Fred noted – and to go left or right, turn the wheel slightly one way or the other. With a bit of practice, Fred reckoned he could give it a go.

All this time, the skipper was totally unaware he was being watched – to him it looked as though Fred was standing there looking straight ahead. In fact Fred was watching his every move with his south-west eye, without needing to turn his head at all! Fred stayed long enough to watch the skipper manoeuvre the boat for the return part of the trip. Having seen enough, he hurried over to where Maisie was sitting so they could compare notes. It was later to be regretted that he didn't stay long enough to see the boat being docked when they got back!

Their next plan of action was to hire a boat. It was all very well for Maisie – she could practise her commentary wherever she liked – but in order for Fred to practise steering a boat, he had to actually do it! With a bit more of their savings (they thought it was worth the investment), they hired a small boat, nothing fancy mind, just something Fred could use for practice. The boat was called *Mistress Maisie*, which they thought was a good omen.

They pulled away smoothly enough, and chugged along happily for a while. Maisie started her commentary, pointing out landmarks to the left and right, while Fred was enjoying the feel of the open water and being the master of the boat.

'This is the life, Maisie me ol' girl. I reckons as 'ow we got a good fing going 'ere.'

Maisie continued her commentary, but soon realised that things she was pointing out to left and right were actually behind or directly in front of them! She wondered what was the trouble?

'Fred,' she cried, 'you gotta keep going straight, you're messing up me commentary!' After all her practice, Maisie was quite upset.

But that was the trouble; because of the orientation of his

eyes, poor Fred couldn't go straight for the simple reason that he couldn't see straight. In order to see straight he would have had to turn sideways on to the wheel, which would have made steering difficult. Consequently, they ended up zig-zagging across the Thames, Maisie having to adapt her commentary as they went, and getting more and more flustered.

They got to the point where they had agreed to turn, and thankfully Fred accomplished this without incident. They zig-zagged back, by which time Maisie had all but given up on her commentary, added to which were loud hoots from other boats trying to go about their business.

They arrived back at the dock. Fred was happy that he had got them there and back safely but Maisie was not happy. At this point, Fred began to regret not having observed how to dock a boat. As they approached the docking area, he didn't have a clue!

It is generally accepted that in order to dock a boat, dock lines have to be prepared on bow and stern, and fenders have to be attached. The approach to the docking area has to be lined up and surveyed. The current, wind, and water conditions have to be judged. The approach to the docking area has to be cautious, using intermittent acceleration.

Fred knew nothing about lines and fenders, it was impossible for him to line anything up, he knew nothing about judging the conditions and he was unable to control the speed of the boat. He simply headed for the docking area and hoped for the best.

The outcome was not a happy one – Maisie was shrieking with fear, and the boat owner was hopping about frantically on the side, waving his fists menacingly. Fred closed his eyes, offered up a quick prayer (the nuns had taught him the power of prayer) and with a thud he met the dock wall port-side on, scraping the side of the boat until it slowly came to a stop.

All hell broke loose. The boat owner was incandescent with

rage – damage would have to be paid for, and Maisie, suffering from fear and shock, was beside herself. Several people came hurrying over to see what all the fuss was about. They alternately tried to console Maisie – 'There, there, pet, you'll be all right' – berate Fred – 'Wha've bloody hell do you fink you're playin' at?' – and sympathise with the boat owner – 'Don't you worry mate, we'll get it fixed for you in no time.'

Mercifully, and Fred only had the Good Lord Above to thank for this, the damage was slight – just a few scratches here and there. Fred thrust the last of his money into the boat owner's hand, and, with all the palaver going on around them, Fred and Maisie crept away. They took stock of the situation, and wisely decided boat trips and guided tours were not for them. Fred could look for other little earners if he wanted to, but Maisie had had enough of little earners; she would look for a proper job elsewhere!

Chapter Five

WEDDED BLISS

Fred was sixteen when he met Maisie and she was just a year younger. They courted for five years until Maisie started dropping hints, and so Fred decided he ought to do the decent thing and propose that they be joined together in Holy Matrimony. For a romantic proposal, it left a lot to be desired; he had just finished cleaning a particularly smelly drain, and so consequently he smelled none too fresh himself! Awkwardly he got down on one knee, looked her lovingly in the eye as best he could, and with an extravagant gesture placed a cheap ring on her finger. Fred never did things by halves, so he had prepared his proposal carefully.

'Well, Maisie me ol' girl, we bin togevver for five years now, and I reckons as 'ow we rub along nicely. I reckons it's about time we got togevver proper like, so I'm asking yer, will yer do me the'onour of being me lawfully wedded trouble an' strife?' (wife, in Cockney rhyming slang). For romantic appeal it had none; for Cockney charm it had plenty!

Maisie accepted gladly, but Fred, being the gentleman he was, thought they ought to see her parents to get their blessings. They were only too pleased – one less mouth to feed – and so gave their blessings readily. Fred had no one to please but himself, so it was all very satisfactory.

The date set was Saturday 21st May 1921. The ceremony was to take place in All Saints, Poplar, followed by a gathering in a local pub. There were plenty to choose from, but in the end the Master's Arms, a third-generation family-run pub, was selected as being everyone's favourite.* A previous landlord had invested in a piano, so a good old knees-up and a sing-song were guaranteed. Frank was Fred's best man and Peggy was Maisie's matron of honour.

The church and pub afterwards were packed, what with Fred being so popular, and Maisie coming from a large family. The nuns provided the food for the wedding feast as their wedding gift and the costers and market traders provided the beer. It was a wedding done in the best Cockney style, and would be remembered long afterwards by friends and family alike. Fred and Maisie had a week's honeymoon in Whitstable.

They rented two small rooms in the bottom half of a small cottage in Cubitt Town, with a yard backing on to the Thames. It was perfect. Fred continued to make money as only he knew how and Maisie, having refused to have anything more to do with Fred's odd jobs or little earners, was quite happy to settle down, keep house and have babies.

A year after they were married the first baby arrived – a boy whom they named Frank, followed two years later by a little girl whom they named Peggy. Over the next few years, they were blessed with four more children – another boy (Ronald), the twins (Winnie and Elsie) and finally little Dorothy. She was the apple of Fred's eye – a tiny wisp of a creature – and everyone called her Dolly for short.

---

* For a full account of the Master's Arms see *Farewell to the East End.*

Chapter Six

HYDE PARK

With more and more mouths to feed, Fred had his work cut out providing for them. He had his regular jobs clearing drains, and attending to the boiler at Nonnatus House, but he needed more money and so he increased his odd jobs and little earners. Once again, he took up some of the suggestions Frank had made a few years earlier, and added window cleaning, office cleaning and a bit of painting and decorating to his list. He bought and sold things, made and sold things, and grew and sold things; there was no end to his inventiveness.

But still it was not enough, and so he decided, with some reluctance, he would have to take up the suggestion Frank had made of collecting manure. He drew the line at dog turds – too smelly and he didn't hold with dogs anyway, having had a nasty experience with one when he was a lad – but horse droppings he reckoned wouldn't be too bad. Maisie wasn't happy, but kept quiet and let him get on with it. After all, he was doing his best, so that the kiddies could have a nice hot dinner on the table.

Fred was blowed if he was going to bend down and pick up horse droppings by hand, so he fashioned an ingenious contraption with which to do so; he used an old crate from the market and removed one side of it, attaching a broom handle to the other side with some nails. Into this the droppings could be scraped, using a broom which had lost all its bristles. It was a marvellous invention, it worked a treat and Fred was immensely proud of it. Nowadays we would call it a pooper scooper; Fred called it his shit shoveller.

Fred caught the bus to Hyde Park, and within a very short time had collected two sacks full of manure, which he planned to sell to the Mudchute allotment holders for six pennies a sack. Horse riding in Hyde Park was popular, and horse droppings were plentiful. Fred reckoned he was on to a nice little earner here!

Fred had given little thought to the return journey, which was unfortunate. He arrived at the bus stop only to be refused entry by the bus conductor.

'Sorry mate, there's no way you're getting on this 'ere bus, with them there sacks full of manure, stinking to high heaven an' all. I got me other passengers to think of, see, an' you'll put them off, what with the smell an' all.'

Poor Fred had no option other than to walk all the way back to Poplar, dragging the heavy sacks with him, a distance of some seven miles!

He trudged along wearily, considering his options; maybe he could get himself a barrow, like what the costers use, but then he'd have to walk there *and* back and that would take even longer. Maybe he should give up the idea altogether, but the thought of a shilling in his pocket, and more to come, was enough to convince him to carry on.

What he needed was a little trolley, small enough to carry there on the bus, but big enough to pull two sacks of manure back. That would be easy enough to make, he thought; all he needed was a fish crate from Billingsgate Market, some old roller-skate wheels, a few nails and a bit of string.

Greatly cheered by this thought, he quickened his step. He'd call in on his mate Spud, who he'd promised the first sacks of manure to. Spud had a plot on the Mudchute allotments and grew prize-winning potatoes. Having delivered the sacks, thus relieving him of his burden, and with a shilling in his pocket, his step was sprightly. The rest of the journey home was no trouble; he was looking forward to seeing Maisie and the kiddies.

PART II

CHUMMY

In which we meet Chummy

When it came to choosing my favourite stories to complement the new material, I just couldn't decide. I think it's fair to say my mother was a natural storyteller and, quite honestly, I was spoilt for choice. Instead, I decided to focus attention on two of my favourite characters: Chummy and Sister Monica Joan. That decision having been made, choosing my favourite stories was then relatively straightforward.

In the following two chapters taken from *Call the Midwife*, we meet Chummy, a student midwife who arrived at Nonnatus House the day after my mother. Dear Chummy, larger than life, awkward, shy and clumsy; a social misfit with a heart of gold. We also meet Cynthia and Trixie, fellow student midwives. Incidentally, Cynthia and my mother remained lifelong friends and Cynthia became my godmother when I was born.

Chapter Seven

CHUMMY

The first time I saw Camilla Fortescue-Cholmeley-Browne, I thought it was a bloke in drag. Six foot two inches tall, with shoulders like a front-row forward and size eleven feet, her parents had spent a fortune trying to make her more feminine, but to no effect.

Chummy and I were new together, and she arrived the morning after the memorable evening when Sister Monica Joan and I had polished off a cake intended for twelve. Cynthia, Trixie and I were leaving the kitchen after breakfast when the front doorbell rang, and this giant in skirts entered. She blinked short-sightedly down at us from behind thick, steel-rimmed glasses and said, in the plummiest voice imaginable, 'Is this Nonnatus House?'

Trixie, who had a waspish tongue, looked out of the door into the street. 'Is there anyone there?' she called, and came back into the hallway, bumping into the stranger.

'Oh, sorry, I didn't notice you,' she said, and made off for the clinical room.

Cynthia stepped forward and greeted the woman with the same exquisite warmth and friendliness that had chased away my thoughts of bolting the night before. 'You must be Camilla.'

'Oh, just call me Chummy.'

'All right then, Chummy, come in and we will find Sister Julienne. Have you had breakfast? I'm sure Mrs B can fix you up with something.'

Chummy picked up her case, took two steps and tripped over the doormat. 'Oh lawks, clumsy me,' she said with a girlish giggle. She bent down to straighten the mat and collided with the hallstand, knocking two coats and three hats on to the floor.

'Frightfully sorry. I'll soon get them,' but Cynthia had already picked them up, fearing the worst.

'Oh thanks, old bean,' said Chummy, with a 'haw-haw'.

Can this be real, or is she putting it on? I thought. But the voice was entirely real, and never changed, nor did the language. It was always 'good show', or 'good egg', or 'what-ho', and, strangely enough, for all her massive size, her voice was soft and sweet. In fact, during the time that I knew her, I realised that everything about Chummy was soft and sweet. Despite her appearance, there was nothing butch about her. She had the nature of a gentle, artless young girl, diffident and shy. She was also pathetically eager to be liked.

The Fortescue-Cholmeley-Brownes were top-drawer county types. Her great-great-grandfather had entered the Indian Civil Service in the 1820s, and the tradition had progressed through the generations. Her father was Governor of Rajasthan (an area the size of Wales), which he still, even in the 1950s, traversed on horseback. All this we learned from the collection of photographs on display in Chummy's room. She was the only girl amongst six brothers. All of them were tall, but unfortunately she was about an inch taller than the rest of the family.

All the children had been educated in England, the boys going to Eton, and Chummy to Roedean. They were placed in the care of guardians in this country, as the mother remained in India with her husband. Apparently Chummy had been at boarding school since she was six years of age, and knew no other life. She clung to her collection of family photographs with touching fervour – perhaps they were the closest she ever got to her family – and particularly loved one taken with her mother when she was about fourteen.

'That was the holiday I had with Mater,' she said proudly, completely unaware of the pathos of her remark.

After Roedean came finishing school in Switzerland, then back to London to the Lucy Clayton Charm School to prepare her for presentation at Court. Those were the days of debutantes, when the daughters of the 'best' families had to 'come out', an expression meaning something quite different today. At that time it meant being presented formally to the monarch at Buckingham Palace. Chummy was presented and two photographs were proof of the event. In the first, an unmistakable Chummy in a ridiculous lacy ball gown, with ribbons and flowers, stood amongst a group of pretty young girls similarly attired, her huge, bony shoulders towering above their heads. The second photo was of her presentation to King George VI. Her great size and angular shape emphasised the petite charm of the Queen and the exquisite beauty of the two princesses, Elizabeth and Margaret. I wondered if Chummy was aware of how absurd she looked in the photos, which she was so pleased about and so happy to display.

After the debutante bit came a year at a Le Cordon Bleu school, which took a small number of select young ladies on a residential basis. Chummy learned all the arts of the perfect hostess – the perfect hors d'oeuvre, the perfect pâté de foie gras – but remained ungainly, awkward, oversized and generally unsuited to hostessing in any society. So a course of study at the best needlework school in London was deemed to be the right thing for her. For two years Chummy crocheted, embroidered and tatted, made lace and quilting and broderie anglaise. For two years she machined and set shoulders and double-hemmed. All to no avail. While the other girls herringboned and feather-stitched and chatted happily, or sadly, of their boyfriends and lovers, Chummy, liked by all but loved by none, remained silent, always the odd chum out.

She never knew how it happened, but suddenly, unsought, she found her vocation: nursing and God. Chummy was going to be a missionary.

In a fever pitch of excitement, she enrolled at the Nightingale School of Nursing at St Thomas's Hospital in London. She was an instant success, and won the Nightingale Prize three years in succession. She adored the work on the wards, feeling for the first time in her life confident and competent, knowing that she was where she should be. Patients loved her, senior staff respected her, junior staff admired her. In spite of her great size she was gentle, with an intuitive understanding of patients, especially the very old, very sick, or dying. Even her clumsiness – a hallmark of earlier years – left her. On the wards she never dropped or broke a thing, never moved awkwardly or crashed into things. All these traits seemed to beset and torment her only in social life, for which she remained wholly ill-adapted.

Of course, young doctors and medical students, ninety per cent of whom were male and always on the lookout for a pretty nurse, made fun of her and passed crude jokes about the difficulty of mounting a carthorse, and which of them had the organ of a stallion suited to the job. Freshmen were told of the ravishingly lovely nurse on North Ward, with whom it would be possible to fix a blind date, but they fled in horror when the blindness was given sight, vowing vengeance upon the jokers. Fortunately, such stories or pranks never reached Chummy's ears and passed straight over her head unnoticed. Had she been informed, it is very likely that she would just not have understood, and would have beamed amiably at her tormentors, shaming them with her innocence.

Chummy's entry into midwifery was less successful, but no less spectacular. It was some days before she could go out on the district. In the first place, no uniform would fit her. 'Never mind, I'll make it,' she said cheerfully. Sister Julienne doubted if there was a pattern available. 'Not to worry, actually I can make it out of newspaper.' To everyone's astonishment, she did. Material was obtained and, in no time at all, a couple of dresses were made.

The bicycle was not so easy. For all the genteel education and ladylike accomplishments, no one had thought it necessary to teach her to ride a bicycle. A horse, yes, but a bicycle, no.

'Never mind, I can learn,' she said cheerfully. Sister Julienne said it was hard for an adult to acquire the skill. 'Not to worry. I can practise,' was her equally exuberant response.

Cynthia, Trixie and I went with her to the bicycle shed and selected the largest – a huge old Raleigh, of about 1910 vintage, made of solid iron with a scooped-out front and high handlebars. The solid tyres were about three inches thick, and there were no gears. The whole contraption weighed about half a ton, and for this reason no one rode it. Trixie oiled the chain and we were ready for the off.

The time was just after lunch. We agreed to push Chummy up and down Leyland Street until she found her balance, after which we would travel in convoy to where the roads were quiet and flat. Most people who have tried to ride a bicycle in adult life for the first time will tell you that it is a terrifying experience. Many will say that it is impossible, and give up. But Chummy was made of sterner stuff. The Makers of the Empire were her forebears, and their blood flowed in her veins. Besides which, she was going to be a missionary, for which it was necessary that she should be a midwife. If she had to ride a bicycle to achieve this, so be it – she would ride the thing.

We pushed her, huge and shaking, shouting 'pedal, pedal, up, down, up, down' until we were exhausted. She weighed about twelve stone of solid bone and muscle, and the bike another six stone, but we kept on pushing. At four o'clock the local school ended, and children came pouring out. About ten of them took over, giving us girls a well-earned rest as they ran along beside and behind, pushing and shouting encouragement.

Several times Chummy fell heavily to the ground. She hit her head on the kerb, and said, 'Not to worry – no brains to hurt.' She cut her leg, and murmured, 'Just a scratch.' She fell heavily on to one arm, and proclaimed, 'I have another.' She was indomitable. We began to respect her. Even the Cockney children, who had seen her as a comic turn, changed their tune. A tough-looking cookie of about twelve, who had been openly jeering at first, now looked solemnly at her with admiration.

The time had come to venture further than Leyland Street. Chummy could balance and she could pedal, so we agreed to half an hour cycling together around the streets. Trixie was in front, Cynthia and I on either side of Chummy, the children running behind, shouting.

We got to the top of Leyland Street and no further. It had not occurred to us to show Chummy how to turn a corner. Trixie turned left, calling 'just follow me', and rode off. Cynthia and I turned left, but Chummy kept going straight ahead; after that, all was confusion. Apparently a policeman had been in the act of crossing the street when she hurtled into him. Seeing a representative of the law hit full frontal by a midwife was joy for the children. They screamed with delight, and doors opened all down the street, emitting even more children and curious adults.

We hastily turned back to see what had happened. I heard a groan, and then the policeman sat up with the words, 'What fool did that?'

I saw Chummy sit up. She had lost her glasses, and peered round. Maybe this could account for her next action, or maybe she was dazed. She slapped the man heavily on the back with her huge hand and said, 'No whingeing, now cheer up, old bean. Stiff upper lip and all that, what?' Clearly she was unaware that he was a policeman.

He was a big man, but not as big as Chummy. He fell forward at the blow, his face hitting one of the bicycles, and he cut his lip. Chummy merely said, 'Oh, just a little scratch. Nothing to make a fuss about, old sport,' and slapped him on the back again.

The policeman was outraged. He took out his notebook and licked his pencil. The children vanished and the street cleared. He looked at Chummy with menace. 'I'll take your name and address. Assaulting a policeman is a serious offence, I'll have you know.'

I swear it was Cynthia's sexy voice that got us off. Without her, we would have been up before the magistrate the next day. I never knew how she did it, and she was quite unconscious of her charm. She said little, but the man's anger quickly vanished, and he was eating out of her hand in no time at all. He picked up the bicycle and escorted us down the street to Nonnatus House. He left us with the words, 'Nice meeting you, young ladies. I hope we meet again sometime.'

Chummy had to spend three days in bed. The doctor said she had delayed shock and mild concussion. She slept for the first thirty-six hours, her temperature raised and pulse erratic. On the fourth day she was able to sit up, and asked what had happened. She was horrified when we told her, and deeply remorseful. As soon as she could go out, her first visit was to the police station to find the constable she had injured. She took with her a box of chocolates and a bottle of whisky.

Chapter Eight

THE BICYCLE

The hidden steel of a Fortescue-Cholmeley-Browne was revealed to us over the next few weeks as Chummy mastered the skills of riding a bicycle. After the accident, Sister Julienne was seriously in doubt as to whether it would be possible, but Chummy was adamant. She could and would learn.

Every spare minute of her time was spent practising. All her district work had to be done on foot in the meantime, and this took far longer than it would have taken on a bicycle. Consequently, she had less spare time than anyone else. But she utilised each and every minute of freedom. She would push the old Raleigh up Leyland Street, a slight incline, and then freewheel down; up and down hundreds of times until she acquired her balance. She got up a couple of hours early each morning, and went out every evening from about eight to ten, coming back exhausted and breathless. 'Well, actually, there's no point in just learning to ride in the daylight,' she argued gaily, with irrefutable logic.

These rides in the dark were usually accompanied by crowds of cheering or jeering children. This might have been a menace, had Chummy not gained the respect of an older lad who had joined us on the first day when Cynthia, Trixie and I had been trying to teach her. Jack was a particularly tough specimen of about thirteen, accustomed to fighting for his rights. He soon dispersed the little kids; a few blows, a few kicks, and they were gone. Then he presented himself in front of the bicycle, her champion.

'You gets any more trouble from that lot, Miss, jes' call me. Jack. I'll take care of 'em.'

'Oh, that's frightfully good of you, Jack. Actually, I'm most awfully grateful. This old machine's a lively little filly, what?'

Chummy's posh voice must have been as incomprehensible to Jack as his Cockney accent was to her, but, nevertheless, they struck a friendship then and there.

After that, Chummy learned rapidly. Jack was out early and late, running, pushing, helping her in every way. He developed a particularly ingenious way of teaching her to steer the bike and turn corners: he pedalled whilst she steered! Chummy controlled the handlebars, sitting on the saddle, her legs trailing, whilst he stood on the pedals, doing all the hard work. To propel her twelve stone weight must have been hard work, but Jack was no puny thirteen-year-old and took pride in his manliness. Early and late he could be heard shouting, 'Turn lef', miss; NO, LEF', yer dafty. Easy does it. Not too sharp; now aim for that phone box, and keep yer eyes on it.'

Neither of them saw defeat as a possibility, and within three weeks they were riding all the way from Bow to the Isle of Dogs in the dark November mornings.

Jack did not own a bicycle, and reluctantly he had to admit that the time had come for Chummy to try on her own. He pushed her off, and she pedalled confidently down the street and round the corner. Sadly he waved as she turned out of sight. He had been useful, and now the fun was all over. He kicked a stone and slouched off homewards, hands in pockets, one foot in the gutter, the other on the kerb.

But Chummy was not one to let a friendship die, still less to allow kindness and help to pass unnoticed. She discussed it with us at lunch, and we agreed that a gift of some sort would be appropriate. Various were the suggestions – a jar of sweets, a football, a penknife – but Chummy was not happy with any of these ideas. Sister Julienne, ever practical and wise, pointed out that the time, effort and commitment on Jack's part had been very great, so therefore her debt to him was great.

'I don't think the boy should be fobbed off with a trivial token. I feel he should receive something that he really wants and would value. On the other hand, it depends entirely upon what you, the giver, can afford, and only you can know this.'

Chummy brightened, and a huge smile lit her features. 'Actually, I know what Jack wants more than anything else – a bicycle! And I'm pretty sure Pater would buy one for him if I explained the circumstances, what-ho. He's a sporting old stick, and always coughs up for a good cause. I'll write to him tonight.'

Of course Pater coughed up, happy to see his only daughter fulfilled at last. He could no more understand her determination to become a missionary than he could understand her passion for midwifery, but he would support it to the end.

A new bicycle meant a new life for Jack. Very few boys had such a possession in those days. For him, it meant more than status; it meant freedom. He was an adventurous boy, and went miles beyond the East End on his bike. He joined the Dagenham Cycling Club and competed in time trials and road races. He went camping alone in the Essex countryside. He went as far as the coast, and saw the sea for the first time.

Chummy was delighted, and his continued friendship was her greatest joy. He seemed to feel she needed his protection, and so, every day after school, Jack would turn up at Nonnatus House to escort her on her evening visits. His instinct that the children of the docks would tease and torment her were right, because, on the whole, the Cockneys did not take to Chummy, and made fun of her behind her back. Her huge size, pedalling steadily along the streets on an ancient solid-wheeled bicycle, brought crowds of children to a standstill, and they lined the pavement shouting things like 'what-ho' and 'jolly good show, actually' or 'steady on, old bean' amid loud-mouthed guffaws.

And, to rub salt into the wound, they called her 'The Hippo'. Poor Chummy treated it with good humour, but we all knew how deeply it hurt her. But when tough, pugnacious, street-wise Jack was with her, the children kept their distance. We all saw him on different occasions, standing in the street or the tenement courtyards, holding two bicycles, his lower jaw thrust forward, his stocky legs slightly apart, coolly looking around him, confident that a look was all that was needed to protect 'Miss'.

Twenty-five years later, a shy young girl called Lady Diana Spencer became engaged to marry Prince Charles, heir to the throne. I saw several film clips of her arriving at various engagements. Each time when the car stopped, the front near-side door would open and her bodyguard would step out and open the rear door for Lady Diana. Then he would stand, jaw thrust forward, legs slightly apart, and look coolly around him at the crowds, a mature Jack, still practising the skills he had acquired in childhood, looking after his lady.

PART III

FRED

In which Fred finds his voice

We return now to the new material. It is the summer of 1957 and Fred decides to embark on a new enterprise. He rather fancies himself as a singer and so he decides to have a go at busking. As with all his little earners, it comes to an abrupt end, and we leave him pondering his next enterprise: toffee apples. This brings us full circle, back to the autumn of 1957, when my mother arrives at Nonnatus House and to the chapter from *Call the Midwife* where we first meet Fred.

Chapter Nine

FRED DECIDES TO BUSK

Of all the unlikely occupations, Fred was once a popular open-air singer. A boiler man, a cleaner of drains and gutters, a small-time entrepreneur buying and selling almost anything legal or illegal; all fitted his character, but a singer? Surely not?

He had none of the glamour associated with a singer, being short and scruffy-looking, with a few grey hairs and one tooth in the centre of his mouth, long and yellowed with age. He looked more like a comic turn than a celebrated singer.

Fred was never without a Woodbine hanging off his lower lip, and he would light a new fag from the remains of the old one. All this raw smoke had been dragged through his vocal chords for forty years, so his voice was husky and gravelly. How, then, could he sing?

With his morning boiler duties at Nonnatus House complete, each Friday Fred would take the bus from Poplar to Tower Hill, north of the Tower of London. Since the Middle Ages, this space has been a meeting place for the citizens of London, both great and good. It used to be a famous hanging ground, and hundreds flocked to watch the spectacle. More recent use has been for public speakers, trying out their fledgling oratory on the heckling crowds.

A bible-waving preacher and a manifesto-waving communist could have pitches next to one another, and each would try and outdo the other. Many people went there for no other purpose than to heckle anyone who had the courage to stand up and have a go. Fridays were the most popular, and lunch-time was the best for all those who wanted a lively audience.

Into this mix Fred would wander, enjoying the crowds, and listening to the multitude of public speakers. Characters the lot of them, Fred thought, all trying to put the world to rights, but all so dreadfully serious. What they needs, he thought to himself, is a lighter touch, then they might get somewhere.

A lighter touch! As soon as the words entered his head, the idea came to him, fully formed. What the crowds needed was entertainers. Politics and strikes and religion were all very well, he thought to himself, but there was no variety. Entertainment was what was needed, and it might just bring in a useful bit of extra bangers and mash (cash, in Cockney rhyming slang). Fred was well pleased with the idea and hurried home to start practising.

He had learned many music hall songs when he was a lad, and when he and Maisie had entertained the people queuing for their tickets, and now he tried to remember them. Many he discarded without further thought as being too rude for mixed company, and he was far too sensitive to risk singing them in front of ladies. But, by trawling his memory, he remembered the words and tunes to a dozen or so.

In the privacy of his back kitchen, he tried them out. They sounded all right to him and he remembered the words – that was the tricky bit, he reckoned – and, with growing confidence, he sang louder. When he got to the sad bits, like poor Molly Malone dying of a fever, he poured his emotion into it until the tears gathered in the corners of his eyes. With the gunfire of 'The British Grenadiers', he stood up straight and assumed a proud military bearing. With 'All the Nice Girls Love a Sailor', he adopted what he thought was a stylish man-about-town attitude, and 'My Ol' Man Said Follow the Van' needed the comic touch so he grinned as he sang.

The more he sang, the more confident he became that the

voice he was hearing was a winner. Nobody had told him that you cannot hear your own voice as others hear it, nor that forty years of heavy smoking would roughen the vocal cords. No one had ever hinted that correct pitch is required to make a tune recognisable, and time, rhythm and correct breathing come into it. Of the finer points of singing he was blissfully unaware, but ignorance, they tell us, is bliss.

Poor Fred had no control over his voice whatsoever, one minute sounding like a foghorn, the next like a screeching cat. In fact, in comparison, he made both of these sound tuneful. He bellowed his songs to the empty kitchen, where the acoustic was good, confirming his suspicion he sounded like Mario Lanza. And why not? Had not the great Italian tenor been discovered in the streets of Naples unloading a truck, singing as he worked, and then been taken to Hollywood to become a star? Fred was realist enough to know he did not look remotely like the handsome tenor, but nevertheless he could sing; he just needed a bit more practice.

If nothing, Fred's vocal range was impressive; he could reach the low notes a Russian Orthodox basso profundo would be proud of, and hit the high notes to rival the best Italian countertenor. The trouble was he couldn't control it, and the transition from one to the other could happen at the most unexpected moments.

One evening he decided to do a bit of practice before bed. As he was belting out 'Molly Malone', a neighbour entered and enquired if everything was all right. 'I thought I 'eard a cat being strangled,' she said. Another neighbour entered the back door. 'I 'eard such a dreadful commotion,' she said. 'It sounded like someone was in pain.'

Fred paused. 'Course everything's all right, ladies. I've never felt better in me life.'

As the two ladies retreated into the street, the noise started again; they looked at each other in alarm. 'Poor man, 'e must be in dreadful pain. My grandad made noises like that passing a kidney stone through 'is you know what.'

The noise stopped and the two ladies looked at each other knowingly. 'He must 'ave passed it,' they agreed, and parted company.

Satisfied with his practice session, and delighted with the impression he had made on the two ladies, Fred went to bed.

Chapter Ten

THE GREAT DAY ARRIVES

Friday dawned bright and clear. Having completed his morning jobs, Fred hurried home to get ready for his debut. The good people of Tower Hill didn't know what was coming! He changed into his old army demob suit (his only suit) and new shoes (blue suede), which he'd bought specially for the occasion. He raked a comb through his thinning hair and brushed his tooth.

Fred's toothbrush had served him well, as he only had the one tooth to brush. In fact, Fred wasn't even sure where it came from, or who had bought it. The toothbrush as we know it today was invented in 1938, so it is possible his dearly departed wife Maisie, ever conscious of the shortcomings of Fred's appearance, had bought it for him before the war.

Fred turned sideways to look in the mirror. 'Gotta look smart,' he said to himself as he adjusted his collar. Satisfied with his appearance, he caught the bus to Tower Hill.

He mingled with the crowds, looking for the best spot to put his soapbox. Ah, there was a good spot. He put the box down and stood on it. Had Fred been tall, or even of average height, he would have looked down on the crowd, but being of such short stature, his eyes were only just level with those of the crowd. Not ideal, but it would have to do. Maybe I'll bring two boxes next time, he thought to himself, as he prepared to launch into his first song.

He pulled himself up straight, puffed up his little chest,

stuck his hand in his waistcoat like Napoleon, and bellowed out:

'I'm 'Enery the eighth I am,
''Enery the eighth I am, I am . . .'

Several people stopped dead in their tracks and stared open-mouthed.

'. . . I got married to the widder next door,
'She's been married seven times before . . .'

'Good God, what the devil is that racket?'

'. . . Everyone was an 'Enery
'She wouldn't 'ave a Willy or a Sam.
'I'm 'er eighth old man, called 'Enery,
''Enery the eighth I am.'

The passers-by were transfixed, scarcely able to believe what they were hearing. Now, it is a law of human nature that when a handful of people stop to look at something, others will join them to find out what they are looking at. Within minutes, four people became twenty, then fifty, then a hundred, all staring in open-mouthed astonishment.

Fred was overjoyed with the crowd. People were leaving the prophets of doom, the trade union bloke and the cruelty-to-animals lady, and coming over to him. He finished his song, bowed to his audience and announced:

'Thank you ladies 'n' gents, thank you. I am now going to sing "Two Lovely Black Eyes".' He cleared his throat, his audience waited expectantly – timing is important – and threw back his head:

'Two lovely black eyes, two lovely black eyes,
'Only fer telling me wife she was wrong, I got two lovely black eyes'

'Put a sock in it, mate,' shouted a voice.

'Give over,' shouted another, 'at least he's trying.'

'Trying me patience more like; give it a rest mate,' joined in a third.

Fred, with majestic composure, ignored the interruption. When the crowd had settled down, he continued:

'*Two lovely black eyes, two lovely black eyes,*

'*Only fer telling the man 'e was wrong, I got two lovely black eyes.*'

'I'll give you two lovely black eyes, mate, if you don't stop,' another voice joined in from the edge of the crowd.

Fred ignored them all and, with a flourish, finished the song.

Thunderous applause; the catcalls and heckling couldn't be heard above the shouts and whistles. Fred continued to entertain the crowd with half a dozen more songs, until he could sing no more. He lit a fag and ambled among the people, holding out his hat.

'He's a fraud, that fella, 'e can't sing.'

'No, but 'e thinks 'e can an' he's got the guts to 'ave a go.'

'He's passing round a hat, bloody cheek.'

'Well, I'm giving him sixpence for giving me a laugh. He's good value for money.'

More people gave money than refused; some patted him on the back. The dispersing crowd were divided in their assessment; some said they had never heard such a dreadful noise, others that he should be supported for having a go. All were agreed he was good comic value.

'Come again,' someone called.

'Right you are, I'll be here next week,' replied Fred.

'So will we be then,' shouted a crowd of office girls.

On the bus ride home, Fred counted out his money. He was astonished: there was more than a month's worth of clearing drains, or raking boilers. This was serious business.

Chapter Eleven

THE END IS NIGH

Every Friday through the long summer months, the political ranters continued ranting and waving their manifestos, the 'end is nigh' preachers continued to wave their Bibles, and Fred continued to entertain the crowds on Tower Hill. Little did Fred or anyone suspect that 'the end is nigh' would come quite as soon as it did.

He had managed to get hold of another soapbox, so the people at the back of the crowd could see him more clearly and he had a greater command of his audience. The only problem was it was a bit wobbly, so he had to be careful getting on it and off it.

Word spread and each week the crowds got bigger and bigger. Newcomers to the scene couldn't believe it and went away puzzled. 'Is he having us on?' was the query in everyone's minds, and they had to come back to satisfy their curiosity.

There have been famous examples of this sort of thing throughout history. At the turn of the twentieth century, a certain Florence Foster Jenkins, a wealthy New York socialite, was convinced she could sing, and every year for a couple of decades she hired the Carnegie Hall to give a 'recital'. Described as the world's worst opera singer, she nonetheless filled the Carnegie Hall and her 'recitals' became a celebrity event in New York.

In 1995, The Really Terrible Orchestra (RTO) was founded in Edinburgh. The orchestra's mission states that: 'The RTO exists to encourage those who have been prevented from

playing music, either through lack of talent or some other factor, to play music in the company of similarly afflicted players.'
The RTO regularly performs to sell-out audiences at the Fringe Festival year after year.

Whatever the precedents, Fred certainly saw himself as a great singer, and he continued to attract large crowds to Tower Hill. He had added some new songs to his repertoire, with miming actions which he had practised in his kitchen.

The crowd cheered when they saw him coming. He stepped up carefully, but nevertheless jauntily, on to his two soapboxes, took a bow and sang:

'There was I, waitin' at the church,
'Waitin' at the church, waitin' at the church;
'When I found he'd left me in the lurch,
'Lor, how it did upset me!'

Fred spread his hands out beseechingly, and the audience sighed in sympathy.

'All at once, he sent me round a note,
'Here's the very note,
'This is wha' he wrote:'

Fred pulled a piece of paper out of his pocket with a flourish and held it up high.

'Can't get away to marry you today,
'Me wife won't let me!'

He let his arms fall in a gesture of despair, and the audience sighed again, deeply moved.

Fred had also been practising a special bow; an attempt at the eighteenth-century courtly flourish. He waved his right arm in a circle above his head, extended his left arm behind him and bowed low at the hips. What with the two boxes being a bit wobbly and Fred's eyes being what they were, he lost his balance and fell off. The crowd roared with laughter, thinking it was part of the act.

With a little assistance, he got to his feet, brushed the dust and bits of mud off his old army demob suit, and tried to assume nonchalance.

'Well, sorry about tha', ladies an' gents. I will now continue.' He launched into a lively rendition of 'Oh! Mister Porter', complete with actions and audience participation. At the end of each verse the crowd joined in with 'What a silly girl I am.'

It had been a good day. Fred lit a fag and started packing away his money, when three men approached him.

'OK, mate, you won't be needing this. We'll take care of it,' and he took the bag of money from Fred.

'Oy! That's mine, just you give it back right now,' Fred cried indignantly.

'You keep your mouth shut and listen to us.' He knocked the fag from Fred's lips and took the packet from him.

The men were big and menacing and Fred felt extremely alarmed.

'I ain't done nothing wrong,' he stammered.

'Nothing wrong! You and yer bloody songs. Here we are, tryin' to whip up support for the cause, an' yer bloody songs are taking away our audience, see.'

'But they likes me songs, it makes 'em happy.'

The man grabbed his shoulders, lifted him clean off his feet and shook him like a dog.

'We don't want 'em happy, see, we wants them to listen to us, to hear wot we 'ave to say about the cause, right?'

By this point, Fred was so scared he was bereft of speech, and could only nod dumbly.

'We see you 'ere again, mate, and it won't be just your money we take, and you'll look a lot uglier than you do now.'

He dropped Fred on the ground, and the three men sauntered off.

The whole episode had taken less than a minute and there were no witnesses. It had been a slick professional job.

For the second time that day, Fred got to his feet, brushed the dust and bits of mud off his old army demob suit, and tried to assume nonchalance, but Fred was seriously shaken and his nonchalance had deserted him.

He was obliged to walk back to Poplar because the money had been taken, so the bus wasn't an option. It was a nice sunny day and, under normal circumstances, Fred would have enjoyed the walk. But not today; he was terrified of meeting the three large men again, and so he fled.

In the small streets close to the river he felt safer, and so he stopped. The river helped calm his state of mind. He sat on one of the sluice gates at Wapping and threw sticks into the water. He felt for his cigarettes but remembered the men had taken them as well. Poor Fred; he felt exceedingly sorry for himself. 'Life just ain't fair,' he muttered, and threw another stick into the water.

Just then, a loud rumble from his tummy and a loud bang from the docks reminded Fred of two things: he was starving hungry, and it would soon be bonfire night. Never one to be down for long, Fred perked up considerably. Dolly, his youngest and his treasure – as she most closely resembled Maisie, with her frizzy hair and cheerful ways – had a nice bit of liver and bacon waiting for him.

As he made his way home to his supper, he recalled with fondness his fireworks enterprise, which sadly the authorities had put an end to (it being a danger to public health), so no hope of making any money that way. There had to be some other way of earning a bit out of bonfire night, and then it came to him in a flash; toffee apples – there had to be good money in toffee apples! He quickened his step as he hurried home to plan his next little earner.

PART IV

CHUMMY

In which Chummy's strength is tested

This chapter is taken from *Farewell to the East End* (the third book in *The Midwife Trilogy*). It is the chapter my father spent hours typing and then inadvertently deleted. The fact that he sat down and typed the whole lot again shows real dedication and the strength of his devotion to my mother. It is a memorable story combining high drama with laugh-out-loud humour; no wonder it is one of my favourite stories. Towards the end we meet again the policeman Chummy crashed into when she was learning to ride her bike.

Chapter Twelve

THE CAPTAIN'S DAUGHTER

It was well that Chummy was on first call. Who else would have had the grit, the stamina and the sheer physical strength and courage to do what she did in the docks that night?

The telephone rang at 11.30 p.m., getting her out of bed.

'Port-of-London-West-India-Docks-nightwatchman speaking. We needs a nurse, or a doctor.'

'What's the matter? An accident at the docks?' asked Chummy.

'No. Woman ill, or somefink.'

'A woman? Are you sure?'

''Course I'm sure. Think I can't tell the difference?'

'No, no. I didn't mean that. No offence, old chap, but women are not allowed in the docks.'

'Well, this one's 'ere all right. Captain's wife or somefink, the mate says. Least, that's what I think he's tryin' 'a say, because he can't speak no English. Just rolls his eyes and groans and rubs 'is tummy – that's why I called the midwives.'

'I'll come. Where do I go to?'

'Main gate. West India.'

'I'll be there in ten minutes.'

Chummy dressed in haste and went out into the night. It was windy. Not cold or raining, but a strong headwind made cycling slow, and it took Chummy nearly twenty minutes to reach West India Dock. The nightwatchman was sitting by the burning brazier next to the gate, which he unlocked.

'You bin a long time. Bloody wind, I s'ppose. Don't like the wind.'

Chummy had never been inside the dock gates before, and the place seemed eerie and alien in the darkness. The stretch of water in the basin looked vast as she gazed down it, and the hulks of huge cargo boats loomed over the oily water. On the skyline, numerous cranes criss-crossed each other. Some of the boats were dimly lit, but others were completely dark. The nightwatchman's coke fire glowed on the quay. The wind caused the water to splash and the rigging to tremble, making hollow moaning sounds.

'Swedish timber carrier on South Quay. Woman got a belly ache or somefink. Shouldn't be there, I told the mate, but I reckons as 'ow he never understood.'

Reluctantly he hauled himself up, left his comfortable little hut and tipped some more coke on to the fire.

'This way,' he sighed mournfully. 'Bloody women. Shouldn't be 'ere, I says. I've go' enough 'a do, wivout all this.'

They made their way to the South Quay.

''Ere we are. The *Katrina*. Yer rope ladder's there and yer guiders.'

He grabbed a rope, pulled it and shouted. A faint sound was heard about forty feet up. The nightwatchman was thinking of his fire, and his cosy hut, and the sausages and fried bread he was going to cook. 'Bloody women,' he muttered, 'no offence to you, nurse.'

A head appeared over the side of the boat.

'*Ya?*'

'The nurse.'

'*Bra. Välkommen. Tack.*'

'Yer'll 'ave to climb the rope ladder. It's leeward o' the wind, an' won't rock too much. You can climb this, can't yer?'

Most women would have taken one look at the bulk of the ship towering above, at the slender rope ladder swinging dizzily in the wind, and said 'No'. But not Chummy.

'Right,' she said, 'Jolly-ho. But I think they will have to haul my bag up separately. I'm not sure I could carry it and climb the ladder one-handed.'

The watchman groaned, but tied the handle of the bag to a rope and shouted to the men above to start hauling. Somehow they understood him, and Chummy watched it swinging upwards.

'Now for it,' she said, taking hold of the rope ladder.

'Ever done this afore?'

'We had a tree house when we were children, so I suppose you could say I've had some practice.'

'The 'ardest part is when you jumps off, because you're goin' to 'it the side of ve boat. But just hold steady and yer'll be all right. Then you can start climbing.'

'Good egg. Thanks for the tip.'

The wind was blowing Chummy's gabardine raincoat in all directions. It was a heavy garment, and long, as required by nursing uniform standards.

'This bally thing's going to be a nuisance.'

She took it off. The nightwatchman looked at her. He was beginning to respect her, and his sausages and fried bread seemed less important.

'Yer skirts too long. You might catch yer foot in 'em.'

'Not to worry.' Chummy pulled her skirt up above her waist and tucked it into her knickers. 'No need for false modesty,' she said cheerily.

She took hold of the ladder again and put a foot on the first rung.

'Go up a rung, so you pull the ladder taut. Grab 'old of a rung above head height. Don't try holdin' the sides of the ladder.'

'Thanks. Any other tips?'

'No. Just keep yer nerve, an' keep climbing. Don't look

down or up. Keep a steady climb, and whatever yer do, don't stop. Jes keep it steady, an' you'll be all right.'

Chummy put one foot on a rung. 'Wizard show, here we go,' she said cheerily, feeling upwards for the next rung. She hauled herself up.

'Only another fifty to go,' she called out to the man watching as she reached upwards for another rung.

'I only 'ope to Christ them Swedes know 'ow to make a rope ladder,' he muttered to himself, 'a weak link could be the death of 'er.'

'What did you say? I couldn't hear for the wind,' she called.

'Nuffink important. Jes' keep going, one hand, one foot. Keep it steady, and don't stop or look down.'

Chummy kept going. The wind was rocking the boat, and every now and then a sudden gust caught her and blew her a few feet to one side. But she kept her nerve. She would have tougher things than this to face when she was a missionary. She remembered Miss Hawkins, a retired missionary and Matron of Queen Charlotte's, where she had done her early training. Matron Hawkins had taught all her students as though they were going to be up a creek without a paddle. Just keep going, old girl, thought Chummy.

She reached upwards and there was nothing. She groped around with her fingers, but no, nothing. Then she felt the wood of a broken rung swinging loose against her arm. Panic hit her and she froze, leaning her head against the side of the ship. To be paralysed with fear can mean death, because the muscles are unable to respond. Chummy listened to her heart pounding and knew her breathing to be shallow and irregular. Her whole body was stiff. She sensed her danger. She was a sensible and highly trained nurse and knew that if she could control her breathing, she would begin to regain control of her muscles. She knew the breathing that she had taught others in antenatal classes would help. Gradually she felt she could move. She brought her foot up to the next rung, which gave her a longer reach, and was able to grab the one above her head with her outstretched hand.

'That was a close shave,' she muttered to herself.

The nightwatchman had seen what had happened, and his heart was in his mouth.

She's got guts, that girl, he thought.

The men above were commenting in Swedish.

Chummy did not know it, but she had not far to go. She felt exhilarated now. Having successfully negotiated the danger of the missing rung, she felt she could tackle anything, and she even enjoyed the rest of the climb. Suddenly she heard voices close to her ear, and her hand touched the metal bars of the bulwarks. She climbed over the edge and stood flushed and breathless on the deck. For once in her life she was not confused or embarrassed to be surrounded by men, even though she was standing among them in her knickers.

'Whoops, cover your legs, old girl,' she said to herself as she let her skirt fall. They all laughed and clapped and cheered.

One of the men handed her the bag then another took her down to a cabin on the middle deck. He knocked and spoke in Swedish. The door opened, and a tall, bearded man appeared. He spoke rapidly to Chummy in Swedish, as though he expected her to understand him. A female voice from within the cabin called out in English, 'Don't try to explain, Dad, I can.'

Chummy entered the cabin, which was very small. A hurricane lamp swung from a hook and the atmosphere was suffocatingly hot. The woman, who was lying on a small bunk bed, was positively huge and not only filled the bunk but spilled out over the edge. She was sweating and dry around the mouth. Her eyes looked gratefully at Chummy. 'Thank God you've come,' she breathed, 'these men will be the death of me.'

The woman lay back and closed her eyes. Heavy blonde hair fell over the grey pillow. Beads of sweat covered her fat features, her chin was indistinguishable from her neck, which in its turn blended into a vast and pendulous bosom.

A small wooden crate in the cabin obviously served as both stool and table. Chummy sat down and took out her notebook.

'I'm glad you can speak English, because I need your case history.'

'My mother was English, my father Swedish. My name is Kirsten Bjorgsen. They call me Kirsty. I am thirty-five.'

'What is your address?'

'The *Katrina*.'

'No, I mean your permanent address.'

'The *Katrina is* my permanent address.'

'That is not possible. This is a trading vessel. It cannot be your permanent home. In any case, I'm told women are not allowed on the ships.'

Kirsty laughed. 'Well, you know, what the eye doesn't see . . .' She laughed again.

'How long have you lived on the boat?'

'Since I was fourteen, when my mother died. We had a home in Stockholm, and I went to school there. But when she died, my father brought me on to the *Katrina*. He is the captain.'

'I was informed that you were the captain's wife.'

'Wife? Who told you that? He's my dad.'

Chummy said no more on the subject, but enquired about the woman's condition.

'Well, I have a pain in my belly. It comes and goes.'

Chummy was beginning to put two and two together. 'When was your last period?'

'I don't know. I don't really take much notice of that.'

'Can't you remember at all?'

'Perhaps a few months. I'm not sure.'

'I need to examine your stomach.'

Chummy palpated the mountainous abdomen, which was all flesh and fat. It was quite impossible for her to tell whether the woman was pregnant or not. She took up her Pinards foetal stethoscope, but it sank about six inches into the abdomen, the flesh virtually covering it, and all that Chummy could hear was the gurgle and swish of intestinal movements.

The woman groaned. 'Ooh, you're hurting me. It's making the pain come back. Please stop.'

But the pain got worse. Chummy felt the lower abdomen and felt a hard round sphere beneath the flesh. When the pain had passed she said, 'Kirsty, you are in labour. Didn't you know you were pregnant?'

Kirsty raised herself on her elbow. 'What?' she demanded, her eyes round and incredulous.

'You are not only pregnant, you are in labour. That's what your stomach pains are.'

'I can't be. You're wrong. I'm always so careful.'

'I'm not wrong.'

Kirsty lay back on the pillow. 'Oh no! What's Dad going to say?' she murmured.

'Which of the men on board is your husband?'

'None of them. And all of them. They are all my boys, and I love them all – well, nearly all, anyway.'

Chummy was shocked.

Kirsty read her thoughts and laughed a great belly laugh, which set all her flesh rippling.

'I'm what you call the "ship's woman". I keep the boys happy. My dad always says there's no fighting on a ship when the boys have a nice woman to go to. That's why he brought me here when Mother died.'

Chummy was deeply shocked.

'You mean to say your father brought you here when you were only fourteen to be . . .' she hesitated '. . . to be the ship's woman?'

Kirsty nodded.

'But that is shocking, disgraceful!' exclaimed Chummy.

'Don't be silly. Of course it's not. After my mother's death, I couldn't stay in Stockholm by myself, and Dad was always at sea. So he took me with him. He explained what was expected of me. He couldn't keep me for himself, because that would cause trouble with the crew – so it had to be fair all round.'

Chummy felt she was choking.

'Your dad explained to you . . . ?' Her voice trailed away.

'Of course. He was always fair, and he still is. But he's the captain, and he always goes first. The other boys have to wait their turn.'

'Your dad goes first?' said Chummy weakly.

'Well, he *is* the captain. It's only right.'

Chummy was thinking about the headmistress of Roedean, and what she would have said about the situation.

Kirsty continued, 'And I never have two at once. Dad wouldn't allow that. He has very high standards.'

'High standards!' Chummy gasped, and the standards enshrined on the coat of arms at Roedean School flashed through her mind – *Honneur aux dignes*, 'Honour to the deserving'. But Kirsty was happily babbling on.

'I love my father, I do. He's a lovely man. He has, how do you say it, the best bugger's grips you've ever seen.'

'Bugger's grips?!' Chummy felt weak from shock. This was a different world.

'You know, whiskers on his cheekbones. They're called bugger's grips. I like to brush them when he's relaxed, after he's done with me. Then he goes to sleep, often. It's like having a baby in my arms.'

Another contraction came, and Chummy sat with her hand on the lower abdomen until it passed. She could scarcely believe what she had heard and needed a few seconds to adjust.

Kirsty chatted on. 'That's better. I feel all right now. I thought it was stomach cramps. I was eating green apples yesterday.'

'No, I assure you. You are in labour and you're going to have a baby.'

'But the boys always wear a rubber when they are doing it.'

'A rubber?' repeated Chummy enquiringly.

'You know – French letters, they call them in England, or *capotes anglaises*, as they say in France. Anyway, the men always wear one. Dad insists, and they wouldn't disobey the captain. And anyway, I make them put one on, or I put it on. Dad gets a great box of them. Five hundred at a time, when we come to a port. He's most particular.'

Chummy felt light-headed.

'Five hundred?' she murmured and stared aghast at Kirsty.

'And they are never reused – Dad insists on that – in case one splits, and I wouldn't know. So you see, I can't be pregnant. It must have been those green apples.'

Chummy couldn't reply to that, but was murmuring, 'Five hundred! How long does a box last you?'

'Oh, a few weeks. Dad would never let me run out. If it's a long voyage, he'll buy in two or three boxes. We always need them.'

'Always?'

'Well, the boys need me, and I'm always here for them. I'm the most important member of the crew, Dad tells me, because I keep the men happy, and happy men work hard. And that's what every captain needs – a hardworking crew.'

Chummy swallowed. She had entered a different world of morality and did not know how to respond.

Kirsty must have read her thoughts because she patted her hand kindly.

'There now. Don't worry. You're only a young girl, and I can see you come from a different class. But it's all quite natural, and I've had a good life. I've travelled the world. Sometimes they can smuggle me ashore and I can have a look round the shops. I like that. I can buy a few pretty things, because Dad gives me money.'

'Don't you do anything else – the cooking, or sewing, or something?'

'Oh no.' Kirsty squawked with laughter and slapped Chummy's shoulder. 'Don't you think I have enough to do with a crew of twenty? Sometimes it's one after another for hours on end. Do you think I could work after that? In any case, we have a ship's cook. He is the one who gave me those green apples yesterday. Oh . . .'

She doubled up with pain. Chummy felt the uterus; it was harder and more prominent. She had timed ten minutes since the last contraction. Labour was progressing.

Chummy had other things to worry about than Kirsty's position on the boat. She was alone, in the middle of the night, on board a ship with no telephone and with a woman in labour. Furthermore the woman was a primigravida of thirty-five, who had had no antenatal care. She should go to hospital at once. But how? In the unlikely event of an ambulance arriving, the woman would be in no condition to climb down the rope ladder! If a doctor was called, would he climb *up* the rope ladder? Chummy remembered her climb, and the missing rung, and knew that she could not expect anyone else to do it. She was alone, and a cold hand gripped her heart. But in the same instant a voice whispered to her that she was going to be a missionary, and that this was just God's way of testing her. She prayed.

The contraction passed, and a new, strengthened Chummy spoke.

'You must stop all this nonsense about green apples. You are in labour, and your baby will be born within the next hour or two. I have to examine you vaginally, and I must have clean cotton sheets, cotton wool and something to act as absorbent pads, a cot to put the baby in, and hot water and soap. Now, where can I get all these things?'

Kirsty looked dumbfounded.

'You must call my father,' she said.

Chummy opened the door and called, 'Hi there!'

The big, bearded man entered, and Kirsty explained. He let out an oath and looked savagely at Chummy, as though it were her fault. But Chummy was taller than him and looked down on him with new-found confidence. The captain turned to go, but Chummy stopped him with a light touch on the arm. She said to Kirsty, 'Would you also tell your father that this cabin is quite unsuitable for the delivery of a baby, and that I will need somewhere better.'

Kirsty translated. The captain no longer looked savage. He looked at Chummy with respect. Then his whole expression changed, and his eyes filled with anguish. He kneeled down beside his daughter, took her huge body in his arms and rubbed his beard into the folds of her neck. He stood up with tears in his eyes and fled from the cabin.

Two more contractions came and went.

They are getting stronger and more regular, thought Chummy. I hope the crew can get something sorted out quickly, because I need to move her, and she has to be able to walk.

The captain returned and said that the best cabin was ready. Kirsty sat up and heaved her great bulk off the bunk. With enormous difficulty, she squeezed herself through the narrow doorway and along the gangways. Several men looked out of their cabins and patted her arms or shoulders. One man gave her a crucifix. They all looked anxious. The ship's woman was not only well used, she was well thought of.

The captain led them to a much larger cabin that was more appropriate in every way. Kirsty gave a cry when she saw it and embraced her father. He kissed her and turned to leave, but first he saluted Chummy in military fashion and bowed to her.

When the door closed, Kirsty said, 'This is the captain's cabin. He's so good to me, I tell you. What other captain would give up his cabin?'

'Well, under the circumstances, and considering he might be the father of the baby, I think it's the least he could do,' retorted Chummy dryly.

The captain's desk and all other naval paraphernalia had been pushed to one side. A large folding bed had been placed in the middle of the cabin, covered with clean blankets and linen. Kirsty looked at it and said, 'I didn't know they had these nice things on board.' A bowl was standing on a small table with jugs of hot water beside it, and soap and clean towels.

Another contraction came, and Kirsty grabbed the edge of the desk and leaned over it. She was panting and sweating. When it passed, she grinned and said, 'You must be right, nurse; this is more than green apples.' She went over to the bed to lie down. 'I still don't know how it happened. I'm so careful. Do you think one of the boys didn't put his rubber on, but told me he had?'

'I don't know. I haven't any experience in your line of business,' said Chummy truthfully, and they both laughed. A bond of female friendship and understanding was developing between them.

Kirsty said, 'You are nice. I'd like you to be my friend. I haven't had any girlfriends since I left school, and I miss them. It's men, men, all the time. I never have the chance to talk to another woman. When I go ashore, which isn't very often, I look at the other women in the streets and think, "I'd like to talk to you and see how you live." But then it's back to the ship and off to sea again.'

'Do the lads ever talk to you?' asked Chummy, who was beginning to sense loneliness.

'Oh yes, some of them tell me all their troubles; they tell me about their wives and girlfriends, and some tell me about their children. It's nice to hear about their children – it makes me feel part of the family.'

Secretly Chummy wondered if the compliment would be returned, but Kirsty was still speaking. 'But I must say most of them just want to be quick and have done with it. I don't mind, if that's what they want, but it's tiring, especially if I get ten or twelve who've only got half an hour before the next shift.' She puffed at the memory. 'You need some strength in my job, I can tell you. These men will be the death of me. Oooh, no, not again!' She threw her body back in pain and cursed in Swedish.

Chummy watched her carefully and made a note that contractions were now coming every seven minutes and lasting for approximately sixty seconds. She could feel the uterus firmly just above the pubic bone, but nothing higher, because abdominal fat occluded it. She longed to be able to hear the foetal heart and reassure herself that the baby was healthy, but it was impossible. She was going to make a vaginal examination. Perhaps that would reveal something. Suddenly she remembered the obligatory enema – that monstrous practice, sacred to midwifery – and abruptly forgot the idea. How absurd on a ship, and surrounded by men! She wrote in her notes: 'Enema not given.'

The pain passed, Kirsty relaxed with a sigh, and Chummy gave her a drink of water.

'I've got to examine you internally,' she said. 'That means I have to put my fingers into your vagina to assess where the baby is lying, and how close to birth it is. Will you allow me to do that?'

'Well, I'm used to that sort of thing, aren't I? But not for the same reasons!'

Chummy placed her delivery bag on the captain's desk and opened it. She scrubbed up and extracted a sterile gown, mask and surgical gloves and put them on. While she was doing so, it occurred to her that Kirsty had probably contracted syphilis during her career. Chummy had no practical experience of venereal disease, but from her classroom work she remembered that syphilis can usually be diagnosed by the hard, rubbery chancre on the vulva, whilst gonorrhoea is manifested by profuse greenish-yellow vaginal discharge. She recalled the midwifery tutor saying that a syphilitic woman very seldom carries to full term, because the foetus usually dies within the first sixteen weeks. She also remembered the next part of the lecture: that in the event of the baby going to full term, it was likely to be stillborn and was frequently macerated. Chummy felt queasy at such an idea. A macerated stillbirth could leave a midwife feeling sick and depressed for days, or even weeks – let alone the effect it had on a mother.

Chummy quickly put the thought from her. Another contraction was coming. She timed it to be seven minutes since the last one. Full dilation of the cervix was getting closer, and as she had been unable to assess the lie of the baby from external palpation, a vaginal assessment was imperative. When the contraction had passed, she said, 'Now I want you to draw your knees up, put your heels together and then let your legs fall apart.'

Kirsty did this with great agility. Her lower limbs were surprisingly flexible. Her massive thighs not only flew apart, but her knees touched the bed on either side, revealing a vast, moist, purple-red vulva. Chummy was a bit taken aback at the speed and efficiency with which the exercise was undertaken, and Kirsty must have seen her expression because she laughed. 'You seem to forget I do this all the time,' she said.

Chummy examined the external vulva carefully. She could neither see nor feel syphilitic chancre, nor was there any evidence of a foul-smelling and profuse vaginal discharge. Against all the odds, it seemed that Kirsty did not have venereal disease. It must have been her father's gifts of boxes of 500 rubbers at frequent intervals that had protected her.

Bully for the captain! thought Chummy.

Chummy did as every good midwife would do. She prepared to place two fingers gently in the vagina, but without the slightest effort her whole hand slid in.

Great Scott! You could get a vegetable marrow in here, she thought.

With easy access she could feel the cervix. It was three-quarters dilated, a head presenting, fairly well down, waters intact. She breathed a sigh of relief that the baby was lying in a good position for a normal delivery.

Then she felt something very strange. At first she thought it was part of the soft, undulating vaginal wall. She moved it with her fingers. It was not part of the vaginal wall.

What on earth is it? she wondered.

It was attached above, and seemed to be hanging freely beside the baby's head. She palpated it with her fingers, and it moved a little. Chummy was feeling this strange thing and moving it about with her fingers, when she realised with horror that it was pulsating. She froze, and blind panic overtook her for the second time that night. She looked at her watch and saw that the thing was pulsating at 120 beats per minute. The pulsation was the baby's heartbeat. The cord had prolapsed.

Chummy said afterwards that in all her professional career she had never known a moment of such terror. She went shivery all over but could feel the sweat pouring out of her body. She withdrew her hand, and it was trembling. Then her whole body began to tremble.

What can I do? she thought frantically. What should I do? Oh please, God, help me!

She nearly sobbed aloud but controlled herself.

'Everything all right?' enquired Kirsty cheerfully.

'Oh, yes, quite all right.'

Chummy's voice sounded far away and faint. She was thinking back to her midwifery lectures: 'In the event of prolapse of the cord, an emergency Caesarean section is necessary.' She looked around the cabin, with the hurricane lamp swinging from the beam; at the portholes, black against the night sky; at the jugs of hot water and towels so thoughtfully provided; at her equipment laid out on the captain's desk, adequate for a normal birth, but no more. The ship moved in the wind, and she remembered her isolation and the impossibility of getting help. She trembled at her own inexperience and thought, 'This baby will die.'

Yet something else was stirring in her mind. The lecturer had not ended with 'an emergency Caesarean section is necessary', but had continued. What else had the lecturer been saying? The pulsating cord, and the knowledge that a living baby depended on her for life, forced Chummy's mind back to the classroom. 'Raise the pelvis by instructing the mother to adopt the genu-pectoral position and sedate the mother. If the amniotic sac is unbroken it is sometimes possible to push the baby's head back a little and move the cord out of the way.'

Good midwifery is a combination of art, science, experience and instinct. It used to be said that it took seven years of practice to make a good midwife. Chummy had everything but experience. She possessed intuition and instinct in abundance. The amniotic sac was not yet broken. There might still be time to attempt the replacement of the cord. She must have a go. She could not sit and do nothing, knowing that the cord would be crushed as labour progressed, and that the baby would die.

'Raise the pelvis,' the lecturer had said. Chummy looked at the massive thighs and buttocks of Kirsty, who probably weighed about thirty-five stone. A crane would be needed to raise her pelvis. The genu-pectoral position would be possible in a smaller woman, but Kirsty could no more roll over on to her front than a beached whale could. But only raising the pelvis would take pressure off the cord, and Chummy was resourceful. She remembered that a folding bed had been provided. If she folded up the legs at the head of the bed, but left the foot end standing, perhaps her patient could lie with her head and shoulders on the floor and her buttocks resting on the higher end of the bed. It was worth a try.

She explained what she wanted to Kirsty. She did not say anything about the cord or the gravity of the situation, because there was no point in alarming her unnecessarily. She merely explained about the bed, as though it was the usual way to deliver a baby.

With great difficulty, Kirsty got to her feet, and Chummy crawled under the bed to collapse the legs so that the head dropped to the floor. That was easy; the difficult part would be getting Kirsty back on to it in the required position. The problem was solved by Kirsty. She calmly went to the raised end of the bed, sat on it, leaned backwards, then rolled her back down the bed. 'I do this all the time,' she said, splaying her legs apart.

Pressure would now be off the cord, Chummy thought with satisfaction – gravity would pull the baby back into the uterus, allowing a little extra space for the cord. But the advantage would not last for long, because the inexorable process of uterine contractions would push the baby forward. Time was short, and running out. Contractions were already coming every six minutes.

Chummy weighed in her mind whether or not to give pethidine to sedate her patient. It would relax her and might help when it came to replacing the cord. But on the other hand it would also sedate the foetus, and delivery was imminent. She decided against sedation. Kirsty seemed relaxed enough and would just have to bear the pain. The life and health of the baby were Chummy's main concern, and pethidine in its bloodstream would be an additional hazard.

A contraction was coming, and Kirsty groaned with pain. She threw her head around and tried to move her legs up to her body.

'Whatever happens, don't roll out of that position, Kirsty. It's perfect,' said Chummy.

I must try to replace the cord before the next contraction, she thought. The time between each would soon be only five minutes.

The contraction passed, and Chummy said a quiet prayer for what she was about to do. She had never seen it done before and had received only one lecture on the subject, but it had to be enough, and with God's help it would be.

'I'm going to push you around a bit, Kirsty. Hook your knees over the edge of the bed, and hold on, so that you don't slip backwards with the pressure.'

Chummy slipped her gloved hand into the vagina. There was no perineal resistance, something she knew she could be thankful for. She felt the partly dilated cervix again, the forewaters protruding and the pulsation of the cord within. With her forefingers she felt around the baby's head – there must be no pressure on the fontanelle, she thought, because that could kill the baby at once. Her fingers were placed, ready to push, when the ship moved, causing them to slip. She had to find the correct position a second time. When she thought her fingers were rightly placed she pushed hard, but the head did not move. She felt the sweat running down her face and neck.

It's got to, she thought. It's got to go back.

So she pushed again. This time the head retreated slightly, but not enough for the cord to be replaced behind it.

After the second unsuccessful attempt, Chummy paused, trembling.

'Pressure, that is the only thing I've got to help me, massive pressure, and God be with me that I do no harm.'

Shaking all over, she leaned her head on the soft cushion of Kirsty's enormous thigh, trying to think clearly. The wind groaned outside, and the ship moved in sympathy. Her fingers slipped and she withdrew her hand. If the amniotic sac broke, that would be the end: nothing could save the baby. Only the fact that the cord was still floating freely in the amniotic fluid made replacement a possibility.

Another contraction came.

Five or six minutes can't have passed, she thought. I can't have spent all that time achieving nothing.

She looked at her watch – it had been five minutes. Contractions were getting closer, and time was rapidly running out.

She saw the uterus heave with the muscular pressure of the contraction, and a plan formed in her mind. Looking at the uterus, her instinct told her that, if she applied reverse pressure externally, and internal pressure on the baby's head, she might be able to move it sufficiently to replace the cord. It was not a procedure that had been taught in the classroom, but something told her that it might work. With only five minutes, perhaps four, before the next contraction, she had to be successful, or the baby would surely die. The ship lurched as a great gust of wind hit the side, and Chummy prayed for calm during the next few minutes.

When the contraction passed, Chummy said, 'Kirsty, I want you to listen carefully. Grip your knees over the edge of the bed again, and hold on. Just concentrate on holding your body still, because I am going to push hard, and you must *not* allow me to push you downwards.'

'I'll do my best, nurse. I have to be strong in my job. I don't suppose you can push any harder than a fifteen-stone first mate. I'll be all right.'

Chummy took her at her word. She inverted her left hand

over the upturned uterus, just above the pubic bone. Being able to insert her whole hand into the vagina was a huge advantage. She cupped the palm of her right hand over the baby's head, stood up and took a deep breath.

'Hold on, Kirsty, don't let yourself slip. I'm going to push – now.'

Chummy was tall and strong. She exerted massive downward pressure internally and externally. The baby shifted two or three inches from her internal hand, but still she kept up the external pressure on the uterus. When she felt it was enough, she relaxed.

'That was hard!' Kirsty said. 'I don't know if I've had it harder than that. But I didn't move, did I?'

Chummy did not reply. Her job was not done. She still had to replace the cord into the uterus. She felt for the cord, but it was not there. She stretched her finger inside the cervical os and ran it around the rim, but could feel only the smooth, round surface of the baby's head. The cord had disappeared. Internal fluid suction, caused by shifting the baby, must have withdrawn the slippery cord without any further action being required from the midwife.

Chummy felt giddy with relief and leaned her head once more on Kirsty's capacious thigh. She giggled weakly.

'It's done, it's done, thanks be to God! And thanks to you, Kirsty. You didn't move. I couldn't have done it without you.'

'All in a day's work,' observed Kirsty casually.

The whole operation had taken only about thirty seconds. But Chummy sat trembling with relief for another two or three minutes, until her more practical side took over. Now that the baby was safe, how was it to be delivered? All sorts of questions tumbled into her mind. Kirsty looked quite comfortable, but could a baby be delivered in an upside-down position? She wondered what the midwifery tutors would say about that! On the other hand, moving this massive female might be a problem. Kirsty had rolled down the slope of the bed, but would she be able to roll up? The third stage of labour, the delivery of the placenta, was vitally important, and Chummy was not confident about the mother expelling a placenta upside down. Kirsty would have to be moved. Then the cord came into her mind. Reverse pressure had made it withdraw into the uterus, but if Kirsty stood up, as she would have to, would the downward pressure displace the cord and make it slip forward again? Chummy could not be sure, but it might. The risk was too great. Kirsty would have to remain in her present position.

Chummy sat beside the labouring woman, listening to the wind and feeling the ship move beneath her. She was not really surprised by the extraordinary situation in which she found herself; after all, she was going to be a missionary and she would have to be prepared for anything. She was a thoughtful, prayerful girl, and she thanked God she was being tested in this way.

She pondered the ugly situation in which Kirsty had been placed. First abused, probably raped, when she was fourteen by her father, and then confined to a ship for the pleasure of all the men, including her father. Yet, Chummy reflected, she seemed happy and content. Perhaps, as she had known no other life, it all seemed quite natural to her. The men were obviously fond of her – their concern as she struggled down the gangway was evident – and she was not ill-treated. Common prostitutes, pushed on to the streets by pimps and beaten up if they protested, had a much worse life, she thought.

Another contraction came, and the waters broke. Thank God I was able to replace the cord, she thought; it was only just in time. Labour was progressing fast, and Kirsty was wonderful. She had had no sedation but had barely murmured at the pain. Chummy could feel the baby's head well down on the pelvic floor. 'It won't be long now,' she said aloud.

Kirsty groaned and pushed. When the contraction had

passed she said, 'I've been thinking about this baby. I'm so glad now. I never thought I'd have one, because Father always gave me the boxes of rubbers and said the boys must always wear them. So they did. But now I'm having a baby. And I'm glad.'

'I'm sure you are. A woman may not want a baby, but she's always happy when it comes,' said Chummy.

'I hope it's a little girl. I'd like a little girl. I have enough men. But I don't want her to have my life. It wouldn't be right for a young girl. I think Father will understand if I talk to him. What's your name, nurse?'

'Camilla,' said Chummy.

'Oh, what a beautiful name. I want to give her your name, nurse, may I?'

'Of course. I should be honoured.'

'Baby Camilla. That's a lovely name.'

Another contraction came, only two minutes after the last, fiercer and longer. Kirsty had no vaginal or perineal resistance, so the head was able to descend quickly and easily. She gripped her hands until the knuckles showed white and pushed hard, forcing the weight of her buttocks against the end of the bed. In protest, the bed trembled and collapsed with a crash on to the floor.

The problem of an upside-down delivery had been solved! Mother and midwife were now on the floor, Kirsty floundering and pushing, Chummy desperately trying to control the situation.

Poor Kirsty was bewildered. 'What happened?' she kept asking.

Chummy, who had narrowly missed having her hands crushed, tried to calm her.

'The bed broke, but the baby is all right, and if you are not hurt, no harm has been done. In fact it's a good thing, because delivery of your baby will be easier.'

*

Chummy's concern now was that the baby's head might be born too quickly. The slow and steady delivery of the head is what every midwife hopes for, but with no perineal resistance, this baby could well shoot out with the next contraction.

Another contraction came, and Kirsty raised her knees and braced herself to push, but Chummy stopped her. 'Don't push, Kirsty, don't push. I know you want to and feel you must, but don't. Your baby's head will be born with this contraction, but I want it to come slowly. The slower the better. Concentrate on *not* pushing. Take little breaths, in-out, in-out, think about breathing, think about relaxing, but don't push.' All the time she was saying these words Chummy was holding the head, trying to prevent it from bursting out of the mother at speed. The contraction was waning, Chummy eased the slack perineum around the presenting crown, and the head was born.

Chummy breathed a sigh of relief. She had been concentrating so hard that she had not noticed the cramp in her legs as she squatted on the deck of the cabin; had not noticed the poor light cast by the hurricane lamp as it swung from a beam; had not noticed the movement of the ship, nor the occasional lurch as the wind hit it. All she knew was that the miracle of a baby's birth would shortly take place, that the safe delivery was in her hands, and that the head had been born. Chummy kept her hand under the baby's face in order to lift it away from the hard floor and waited. Another contraction was coming. Chummy felt the face she was holding move.

'It's coming, Kirsty. You can push now. Hard.'

Kirsty drew her legs upwards and pushed. Chummy eased the shoulder out and downwards. The other shoulder and arm quickly followed, and the whole body slid out effortlessly.

'You have a little girl, Kirsty.'

Emotion flooded over Kirsty with such intensity that she could not speak. Tears took the place of words. 'Let me have her. Can I see her?' she spluttered, still floundering with her head on the deck, unable to lift her shoulders.

Chummy said, 'I am going to lay her on your tummy while I cut the cord, then you can hold her in your arms.'

The baby sank into the soft cushion of her mother's stomach. She was slightly blue around the mouth and extremities, but otherwise she seemed to have suffered no harm from the drama of labour. Chummy severed the cord and then held the baby upside down by the heels. Kirsty gasped and held up her hands protectively.

'Don't worry, I'm not going to drop her,' said Chummy. 'This is done in order to drain the mucus out of the throat, and to help breathing.'

Then she gave a short, sharp pat to the back of the baby, who at once gave a shrill yell. 'That's what I like to hear, let's have another one.' The baby obliged, crying lustily, and from outside the door a chorus of men's voices were heard cheering, shouting, whooping and whistling. They started to sing, in a united and raucous male voice. Kirsty called out to them in Swedish, but they were making so much noise they could not hear her. The captain's daughter was obviously very popular, and the men responded in their own way. 'I expect they will all get drunk now,' she said dryly.

Chummy wrapped the baby in a towel and placed her in the arms of her mother, who was weeping with joy. 'Are you all right on the floor like that?' Chummy enquired with concern.

'I've never been better in my life,' answered Kirsty. 'I would like to stay here for ever, cuddling my baby.' She gave a sigh of contentment.

Chummy now had to deal with the third stage of labour. In retrospect she would say that it was not the most comfortable third stage she had conducted, sprawled as she was across the floor, but at least it was uneventful.

Chummy washed Kirsty and cleared up the mess as best she could under the circumstances. The problem of how to get Kirsty up off the floor was her next concern. The mother obviously couldn't care less. She was cuddling, and cooing, and whispering sweet nothings to her baby. Calling the captain was Chummy's only option, but Kirsty was stark naked. Chummy's modesty shrank from the thought of exposing her patient, naked, to a crowd of men, until she remembered Kirsty's profession. She explained to Kirsty that help was needed and opened the door.

A dozen or more bearded faces appeared at the door, all peering in. At once they started cheering and clapping again. Chummy beckoned to the captain, who strode in, shutting the door behind him. She indicated what was necessary, and he nodded. She took the baby from her mother and retired to a stool in the corner.

The captain was a big man, and strong, but for sheer body weight his daughter could easily have doubled him. He took both of her hands and pulled – the bulk shifted a few inches. He stood astride her body and pulled again; no result. He went to the door, shouted, 'Olaf, Bjorg!' and two massive men entered. He explained, and they nodded. He took her hands again, and one man stood behind each shoulder. As the captain pulled, each man heaved until Kirsty was sitting upright. They gave a cheer. This is obscene, Chummy thought; I can't bear to look at that poor woman sitting there with her huge breasts swinging on the floor, and these men cheering. They were obviously debating how to get Kirsty on to a chair. The debate was long and contentious; each man had his own ideas. A chair was solemnly brought forward and placed behind the woman. The three men grabbed her torso and heaved once more.

That's not the way to do it, thought Chummy, who had been taught how to lift a heavy patient. You'll never get her up like that.

They didn't. After another debate, they tried again, the two men locking their arms under Kirsty's armpits and the captain ready with the chair.

That's more like it, thought Chummy.

I have said that Chummy had cleared up the mess as best she could under the circumstances. But resources were minimal, and the deck of the cabin was still slippery in patches.

The two men lifting Kirsty nodded to each other, took a deep breath and heaved. Her bottom lifted about six inches from the deck. Olaf, on her left, moved his foot and trod on a slippery patch. He hurtled forward across Kirsty's body and Bjorg was thrown backwards. In his fall he flung his arm upwards and hit the hurricane lamp with such force that it shattered, plunging the cabin into darkness.

In the meantime Kirsty had acted. A desperate mother can do anything in defence of her child. As the lamp shattered she screamed, 'My baby,' pushed Olaf, who was lying sprawled over her, to one side, scrambled to her feet, and ran over to the corner where Chummy was sitting. She took the baby, enfolding her protectively to her bosom. When another hurricane lamp was brought in, she could be seen by all the men sitting quietly on a chair, rocking her baby, with a sheet modestly draped around her.

When the cabin was cleared of men, Chummy set about making it into a suitable lying-in room for mother and baby. The bed was not broken, the legs had merely folded in on themselves, so she fixed it up again for Kirsty. But there was no clean linen left after delivery, and her patient had no nightie. There was no cot for the baby, no means of bathing her, and no clothes for her. She explained her needs to Kirsty, who was not really listening, so she went to the door, opened it, and shouted, 'Olaf!' The biggest of the bruisers entered and stood to attention, looking ill at ease.

'Tell him I need more clean linen, two more pillows, some

nightdresses and a dressing gown for you. Also I need some more hot water and more clean towels for me to bath the baby; a box or basket which I can make into a cot, and some soft linen or cloth that I can tear up and make into cot blankets.' She considered there was no point in asking for baby clothes.

Kirsty translated, and Olaf looked mesmerised. She repeated the instructions two or three times, and Chummy could see him desperately trying to activate his brain and memorise the list, which he was counting off on his fingers. He left the cabin, and Chummy set about clearing things up a little more and packing her delivery bag. She was beginning to feel tired. The drama of the night had kept the adrenalin pumping through her body, but now that all danger for mother and baby had passed, her limbs felt heavy and slow.

Olaf reappeared with an armful of stuff, and a second man brought in a jug of hot water. Chummy was able to bath the baby, with Kirsty eagerly watching and commenting at every stage. A basket, which smelled of fish, had been provided, and this Chummy transformed into a crib. She made up the bed with clean linen – but still there was no nightie. Chummy could not allow her patient to remain naked, so summoned Olaf again.

Kirsty explained what was wanted, and the man turned bright red. How very extraordinary, thought Chummy, that this man, who has regularly been having intercourse with this woman, should be embarrassed to have to fetch her a nightie!

He went away and came back with a bag full of women's clothing, which he handed to Chummy without looking at her.

Breastfeeding was the next thing for Chummy to think about. One really wants to establish breastfeeding immediately after delivery and ensure that the colostrum is flowing and that the mother has, at least, a vague idea of what she should do. Kirsty's breasts were so huge that they rested on the bed on either side of her. The baby could easily be suffocated by these mammoth mammaries, Chummy thought, as she expressed some colostrum. She tried the baby at the breast, and the child, surprisingly, opened her mouth, latched on and sucked vigorously a few times. Kirsty was in an ecstasy of delight. Flushed, with sparkling eyes and radiant features, she looked quite different. She must have been a pretty young girl, thought Chummy, before she became the inert, sexually active queen bee in this hive of males.

By now, Chummy was so tired that she could scarcely stand. She sat down on a chair beside Kirsty, who was examining the baby's fingers and toes.

'Look. She has little fingernails. Aren't they sweet? Like little shells. And I think she's going to have dark hair – her eyelashes are dark, have you noticed?' Kirsty looked up. 'Are you all right, nurse? You don't look too good.'

Chummy muttered, 'I'll be all right. Do you think someone might bring us a cup of tea? You could do with a cup also.'

Kirsty called out, and Olaf entered. She gave her instructions, and five minutes later he reappeared carrying a tray laden with good food and fresh coffee. He placed it on the captain's desk and then, rather sheepishly, took a quick look at the baby and sidled out.

'Did you see that?' said Kirsty incredulously. 'They're treating me like a lady.'

Chummy poured the coffee. The caffeine perked her up a bit, and she began to feel stronger. She knew that she would need to, because one more task faced her. She had to get down the rope ladder. She had another cup of coffee and a sweet pastry, which gave her some energy. She left, telling Kirsty that she would return later in the morning.

Up on deck, the dawn was breaking. The wind had dropped, and thin shafts of red-gold sunlight filtered through the grey clouds. Seagulls were swooping and squawking. The docks looked beautiful in the half-light, and the fresh, cold air stung her cheeks. One of the men was carrying her bag, and they all clustered around, cheering and clapping. Chummy walked to the side and looked over the edge. It looked a long, long way down, and the rope ladder looked flimsy. If I can do it once, I can do it again, she said to herself, putting her foot on the rail. Then she remembered her skirt, and the danger it presented. So without any inhibition – she who was chronically inhibited in the presence of men – she pulled it up, tucked it into her knickers and climbed over the side. Her main anxiety was the missing rung, but she knew roughly where it was, and was prepared for the gap. When it came, it was not as hard to negotiate as she had expected, and with a sigh of relief she continued to the quayside. One of the men tied her bag to a rope and let it down for her. She untied it, released her skirt, waved to the men above, and set out for the dock gates, her body tired, but her whole being exhilarated with the joy of having successfully delivered a healthy baby to an eager and loving mother.

The nightwatchman was preparing to go home for the day. He collected his supper box, put away his frying pan, doused his fire and was sorting out the key to lock his hut when two policemen approached the dock gates.

'Morning, nightwatchman. Fair morning after the storm.'

The nightwatchman turned. His fingers were stiff, and he was fumbling with the key, unable to find the keyhole.

'Dratted key,' he muttered. 'Fair morning? Fair enough. Don't like the wind.'

'Quiet night for you?'

'Quiet enough. Would 'ave been quiet, 'cept for bloody women gettin' in the way.'

'Women?'

'Yes, women. Shouldn't be 'ere, I say.'

The policemen looked at each other. They knew that the

Port of London Authority was very strict on women entering the docks, especially since the previous year when a prostitute had slipped in the dark from a gangplank and drowned.

'Which vessel?' The policeman took out his notebook and pencil.

'The *Katrina*. Swedish timber merchant.'

'Did you see the women?'

'Saw one of 'em. A nurse. Her bicycle's over there. Don't know what to do wiv it. An' 'er coat an' all. Don't know what to do wiv it, neither.'

'A nurse?'

'Yes. Woman ill on the *Katrina*, so I calls the Sisters, and a nurse comes.'

'You had better tell us what happened.'

'About eleven thirty. A deck hand, 'e comes to me, saying, "Woman, woman", rollin' his eyes an' rubbin' 'is stomach, an' groanin'. So I calls a doctor, but 'e's out, so I calls the Sisters, an' a big lanky nurse comes, an' I takes her to the *Katrina*, South Quay. Right plucky girl, she was. Climbs up the rope ladder an' all.'

'What! A nurse climbed the ship's ladder in that wind?'

'I'm tellin' yer, big plucky girl. Climbed up, she did. And a rung was missing near the top, an' all. I saw it wiv me own eyes, I did.'

'Are you sure?'

'Course I'm bleedin' sure. Think I'm bloody daft?' The nightwatchman was offended.

'No, of course not. What happened next?'

'Search me. She climbed on board, an' she's still there, for all I knows. Leastways she hasn't collected 'er bike, nor 'er coat, neiver.'

The two policemen conferred. This was a matter for the Port of London Police. The Metropolitan had no authority inside the ports. But was it true? Nightwatchmen, due perhaps to their solitary calling in the darkest hours, were known to fantasise.

The man was fumbling with his key again. He turned and glanced down the quay. 'There she is. That's 'er. Told yer, didn't I? Big lanky girl.'

The two policemen saw a female figure wandering towards them. Her footsteps were uncertain, and she staggered rather than walked. The ordeal of climbing down the rope ladder had taken the last reserve of Chummy's strength. One of the policemen stepped forward to meet her and took her arm. She leaned on him heavily, murmuring, 'Thank you.'

He said, 'Haven't we met somewhere before?'

She looked at him vaguely. 'I'm not sure. Have we?'

He smiled. 'It doesn't matter.'

She walked towards her bike.

He said, 'I don't wish to be rude, nurse, but are you fit to ride a bike?'

She looked round and slowly gathered her thoughts.

'I'll be all right. I must admit I feel a bit queer, but I'll be all right.'

The bike was a big, heavy Raleigh, iron-framed and ancient. She took hold of the handlebars, but it felt so heavy she could barely move it.

The policeman said, 'Nurse, I really do not think you should ride that cycle, especially down the East India Dock Road just as the ports are opening and the lorries are coming in. In fact, in the name of the law, I am telling you *not* to ride it. I am going to call a taxi.'

'What about my bike?' she protested. 'It can't stay here.'

'Don't worry about that. I will ride it back for you. You are going to Nonnatus House, I think. I know where it is.'

In the snug comfort of a London taxi, Chummy fell sound asleep. She was confused and barely articulate on waking, so the driver had to help her out and then rang the bell for her. The

Sisters were just leaving the chapel when it sounded. Novice Ruth opened the door to see a cab driver supporting Chummy and holding her bag. Her first reaction was to think that the nurse was drunk. 'Sit down here,' she said to Chummy. 'I'll fetch Sister Julienne.'

Sister Julienne came quickly, paid the cab driver and turned her attention to Chummy, who seemed unable to move.

'What is the matter, my dear?' She did not smell of drink. 'What has happened to you?' Perhaps she had been beaten up.

Chummy mumbled, 'I'm all right. Just feel a bit funny, that's all. Don't worry about me.'

'But what happened?'

'A baby.'

'But we deliver babies all the time. What else happened?'

'On a ship.'

'A ship! Where?'

'In the docks.'

'But we never go into the docks.'

'I did. I had to.'

'I don't understand.'

'The baby was born there.'

'You mean that a baby was born on a merchant vessel?'

'Yes.'

'How extraordinary,' exclaimed Sister Julienne. 'This requires further investigation. Do you know the name of the ship?'

'Yes. The *Katrina*.'

'I think you had better go to bed, nurse. You don't look yourself. Someone else can clean and sterilise your equipment. I must take your record of the delivery and look into this.'

Chummy was helped upstairs to her room, and Sister Julienne took the midwife's record to her office to study. She could scarcely believe what she read. She rang the doctor, and they agreed that they must examine the mother and baby on board the ship and have them transferred to a maternity hospital for proper postnatal care.

They met at 10 a.m. at the gates of the West India Docks. Sister looked very small and out of place. She explained to the porter that they must go aboard the *Katrina*, where a baby had been born during the night. He looked at her as though she were mad, but said that he would inform the harbour master.

A short time elapsed, and the harbour master arrived with the docking book in his hand. A berth had been reserved for the *Katrina* for three more days, but she had pulled anchor and sailed at 8 a.m.

Sister was horrified. 'But they can't do that. There is a mother and baby on board, just delivered. They will need medical attention. It's the height of irresponsibility. That poor woman.'

The harbour master gave her a very dubious look, and simply said, 'Women are not permitted in the docks. Now, excuse me, but I must ask you to leave.'

Sister would probably have said more, but the doctor led her away.

'There is nothing you can do, Sister. They have gone, and if the captain has done a runner, frankly, I am not surprised. A ship's woman, as they are called, contravenes all international shipping laws. If a mother and baby were found on board, the captain would be arrested. He would certainly be dismissed from service, he would be heavily fined and might have to face a prison sentence. It is no surprise that he left port three days ahead of schedule. By now, the *Katrina* will be well out in the English Channel.'

PART V

SISTER MONICA JOAN

In which we meet Sister Monica Joan

When my mother arrived in the East End of London to start part two of her midwifery training, she didn't know what had hit her. When Sister Monica Joan answered the door of Nonnatus House, my mother nearly ran a mile. Coming from rural Buckinghamshire, she had never seen anything like the slum dwellings of the East End. She had no idea Nonnatus House was a convent, so to be greeted by this tall, angular, elderly nun, dressed from head to toe in full monastic habit, was a terrible shock. It was only the appearance of Cynthia coming down the stairs, dressed in her nurse's uniform, that reassured my mother that, against all the odds, she was indeed in the right place.

Sister Monica Joan – intelligent, highly eccentric, wilful and on occasion downright rude – fascinated my mother and they formed a close and enduring bond. Her stories appear right across the trilogy and choosing my favourites were difficult. These two chapters are taken from *Farewell to the East End*. The opening paragraph refers back to the shoplifting episode, which can be found in full in *Shadows of the Workhouse* (the second book in *The Midwife Trilogy*).

We meet again Mrs B, who loved Sister Monica Joan unconditionally, and Fred, the polar opposite to Sister Monica Joan in every respect. When Fred and Sister crossed paths, the consequences were often hilarious. These chapters conclude Sister Monica Joan's story.

Chapter Thirteen

THE ANGELS

While she could vividly remember things from long past, Sister Monica Joan's short-term memory seemed to be getting shorter and shorter. She appeared to have completely forgotten the unpalatable fact that she had been before the Court of the London Quarter Sessions on a charge of larceny only a few months previously. The prosecution had alleged that she had stolen jewels from Hatton Garden and initially all the evidence had pointed to her guilt. But a surprise witness proved her innocence. The trial had been a shock, to say the very least, for the convent, but for Sister Monica Joan it was as though it had never happened. She was her old self, delightful and entertaining in her conversation, but in her behaviour she was becoming increasingly eccentric and unpredictable.

Sister had a niece, more accurately a great-niece, living in Sonning, Berkshire. They had not met or communicated for many years. One day, Sister decided to visit her niece, and, what is more, she determined that a pair of fine Chippendale chairs, which she had in her room, should be presented to the woman as a gift. Accordingly, she left Nonnatus House early one morning while the Sisters were at prayer, and before Mrs B the cook or Fred the boiler man arrived. How she carried two chairs downstairs is impossible to conjecture, but she did.

Out in the street, she carried one chair to the corner and then came back for the other. She proceeded in this fashion to the East India Dock Road, where a policeman approached and asked her if he could help. Sister Monica Joan did not like policemen. She exclaimed, 'Tush, out of my way, fellow,' and rammed the chair leg into his stomach. The policeman decided to let her get on with it.

Sister reached the bus stop and sat down to regain her breath. A bus came, and the conductor, being a kindly soul, helped her on with her two chairs and put them in the luggage hold. When they reached Aldgate, he helped her off and pointed to where she could catch a bus to Euston, where she would have to change on to another for Paddington station.

It was approaching rush hour when the bus trundled into Paddington. The bus stop was some distance from the railway station, so Sister left one of the chairs (being Chippendale, of enormous value) at the bus stop whilst she carried the other to the station. Then she left that one in the station forecourt and returned for the second. Once in the station, things became easier for Sister Monica Joan, because she found a porter who loaded the chairs on to his trolley and took them to the train bound for Reading, where she would have to change on to a branch line for Sonning.

Meanwhile, at Nonnatus House the alarm was raised. Sister Monica Joan was missing, and no one had a clue where she had got to. Mrs B was in tears. The police were informed but could offer no help. At lunchtime, a phone call was received stating that a policeman had reported seeing a nun at six o'clock in the morning in the East India Dock Road, and that she had rammed a chair leg into his stomach.

'A chair leg!' cried Sister Julienne incredulously. 'What was she doing with a chair leg?'

'She was carrying a chair,' replied the duty policeman.

'But that's impossible. She is ninety, and it was in the East India Dock Road, you tell me?'

'I'm only telling you what the constable reported, ma'am. I'm not making anything up. Now, if you will excuse me, I have work to do. We'll keep an eye open for this missing nun, and if we have any more reports of her activities, you will be informed. Good day to you, ma'am.'

Sister went hastily to Sister Monica Joan's room and observed that not only one chair was missing, but two! Lunchtime conversation around the big dining table focused on nothing else, and prayers were said for Sister Monica Joan's safety.

The train reached Sonning station at about midday, and Sister Monica Joan telephoned her niece. There was no reply. So she decided to go with God and sat down on one of the chairs to have a little doze. A kindly porteress gave her a cup of tea. At about four o'clock she telephoned again, and this time she was lucky. Her niece was at home. Her astonishment at hearing from her great-aunt after so many years, especially as she was waiting at the station with two chairs, can only be imagined. The niece came in her car to collect her aunt. Only one chair could be fitted into the boot, so the other had to be left on the pavement outside the station. It was still there when she returned a couple of hours later.

They telephoned the convent at about five o'clock. The niece said her aunt was tired but happy, and was welcome to stay for a few days if she wanted to. She added that she had received no warning of the intended visit, and that it was only by chance that she was at home at all, as her work often took her away for several days at a time. What would have happened to her aunt had she been away, she could not imagine. The telephone was passed to Sister Monica Joan, who in reply to Sister Julienne's anxious enquiries said, 'Of course I'm all right. Don't fuss so. Why should I not be all right? The angels look after me.'

The angels certainly had a heavy responsibility looking after Sister Monica Joan, and they could never relax their vigilance for a moment. Take the occasion when she nearly set fire to herself, for example. She had complained that the light in her room was insufficient, and that she could not see to read in bed; it was not good enough, something must be done. Obligingly, Fred ran a small cable up the wall and fixed a light just above her head. It was nothing fancy – just a bulb over which a small, fringed shade was placed. Sister Monica Joan was delighted. So simple; dear Fred – she could always rely on him, and now she could read in bed all night if she wanted to.

She did want to, with alarming consequences. Since her bout of pneumonia, caused by wandering down the East India Dock Road in her nightie on a cold November morning, Sister Monica Joan had been favoured by being allowed to have her breakfast in bed. Mrs B usually took it up around 9 a.m., after we midwives and nurses had gone out on our morning visits. But the angels must have seen to it that Mrs B needed to be at the market by 9 a.m. that particular morning, and so she took Sister's breakfast up at 8 a.m. We were all in the kitchen having our breakfast, and the nuns were still in chapel. The House was quiet, except for the scratch-scratch of Fred raking out the boiler. A piercing scream, followed by louder repeated screams, shattered the calm. We girls and Fred rushed into the hallway, all shouting, 'What is it, where did it come from?' The chapel door opened, and the nuns ran out. (Nuns have been known to run, when the occasion demands!) The screams had stopped, but we could hear someone rushing about on the first floor. 'Stay where you are,' ordered Sister Julienne. 'Fred, come with me.' Disappointed at missing the drama, I waited with the others in the hallway. A smell of burning now filled the air. More running feet, more muffled voices, and smoke billowed along the corridor. Someone went to the bathroom, taps were turned on, windows were closed, banging and stamping was heard, and then Sister Julienne's calm voice: 'I think we have got it under control now. Thank God you came up when you did, Mrs B, otherwise I tremble to think of the outcome.'

Sister Monica Joan, protesting about being disturbed, was

led out of her room and away from the smoke to the safety of the ground floor. Mrs B was in a very much worse state. She was pale and shaking, and needed several cups of strong tea fortified with whisky before she could tell us what had happened. Sister had had her new light on, with the pillows arranged so that she could sit up. The topmost pillow was touching the light bulb, and she must have fallen asleep. As Mrs B entered the room, a tiny flicker of flame no more than an inch high had leaped from the pillow. Mrs B screamed and dragged it from under the sleeping head. The open door and the movement had caused the pillow, which must have been smouldering for some time, to burst into flames. Her repeated screams brought help, and a rug thrown over the burning pillow and heavy stamping had controlled the fire. But the smoke was terrible, and they were lucky not to have been overcome by fumes. In the meantime, Sister Monica Joan had sat on the bed saying, 'Gracious heaven! What *are* you doing?'

No one was hurt. The hem of Sister Julienne's habit was badly scorched, but she was not burned. They were all black with smoke and soot. But Sister Monica Joan was the least troubled of anyone. Either she genuinely forgot about it or decided that it would be expedient to do so (I could never be quite sure), but she did not refer to the incident again. When the light was removed from above her bed she said nothing, but she put on her hard-done-by look.

Then there was the occasion when Sister Monica Joan got stuck in the bath. We girls first became aware that something was amiss when we heard movements and voices from the Sisters' floor during the period of the Greater Silence. This is the time after Compline, the last office of the day, and before Mass, the first of the new day, during which complete silence is observed in the monastic tradition. But on this occasion, the Sisters were by no means observing the rule. First we heard one or two whispered words, then more, then a gaggle of anxious voices all talking at once, accompanied by banging on a door, and calls of 'Sister, can you hear us? Open the door.'

What was going on? We looked enquiringly at each other. Novice Ruth came running downstairs.

'Is Fred still here? Has he gone yet?' she called as she ran towards the kitchen. We didn't know, but then heard, 'Fred, thank goodness you are still here. Come quickly to the second floor. We think you'll have to break down a door.'

Mysterious! Exciting! Thrilling! We girls looked at each other expecting more.

We heard more voices upstairs but didn't know what was going on. Fred came back down and passed us as we stood expectantly on the landing.

'What is it, Fred? What's up?'

'I'm goin' outside to see if the winder's open.'

'The window? We thought it was a door.'

'It'll be easier.'

'Than what?'

'Than breaking the door.'

And off he ran.

At this point, Sister Julienne came downstairs and met Fred coming in.

'Yes, Sister. Winder's open. I reckons as 'ow I can do it.'

'Oh, Fred, you're wonderful. But do be careful.'

Fred assumed an heroic air.

'Don' choo worry 'bout me, Sister. I'm OK. We gotter ge' the ol' lady safe, like. I'll get the ladders.'

And off he ran.

Cynthia spoke. 'Sister, please tell us what is going on.'

'Well, the bathroom door is locked. It seems that Sister Monica Joan is in the bath and can't get out, but no one can get in to help her.'

Eager to get a slice of the action, I said, 'Fred's getting on

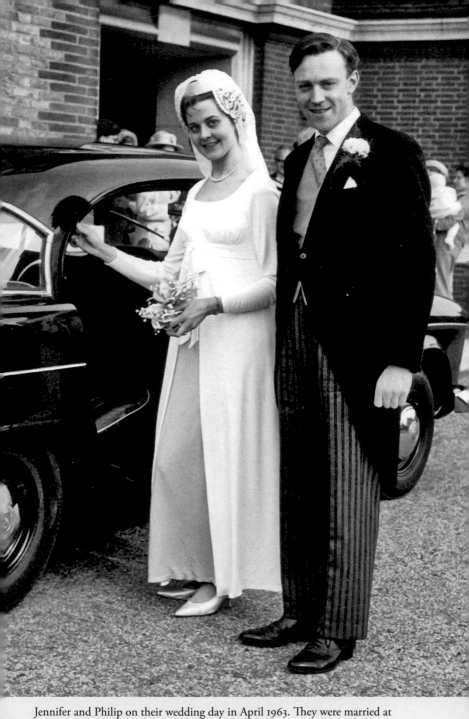

Jennifer and Philip on their wedding day in April 1963. They were married at
St Jude's on the Hill in Hampstead Garden Suburb.

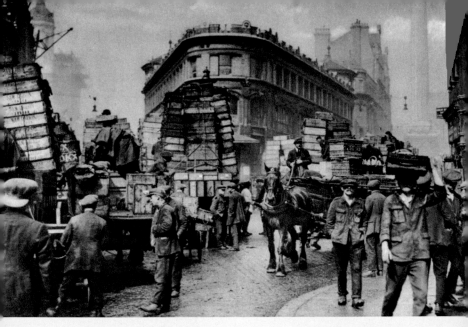

Fish porters in Billingsgate Fish Market, around 1920, where Fred met
Frank. The boxes of fish were stacked high on the carts and barrows,
sometimes on top of the porters' heads.

Interior of a wash house, similar to the one where Maisie worked.

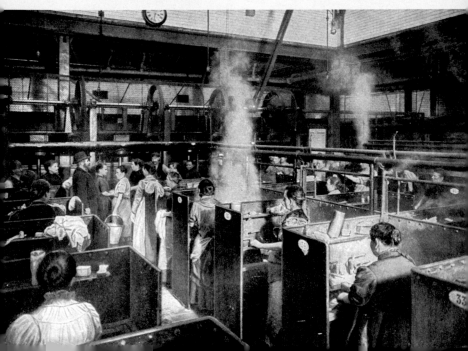

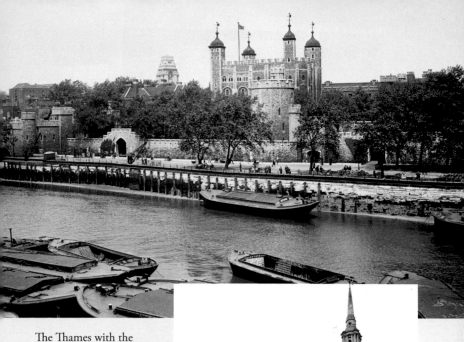

The Thames with the Tower of London in the background, around 1920. The scene of one of Fred's less successful 'little earners'.

All Saints Church Poplar, where Fred and Maisie got married.

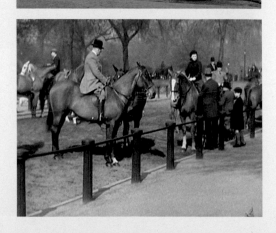

People riding horses on Rotten Row, Hyde Park, around 1930. The scene of a more successful 'little earner'.

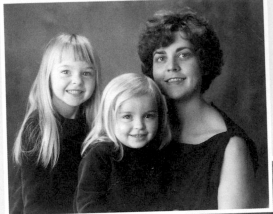

Jennifer with her daughters: Suzannah (left) and Juliette (right) in 1968. We were all wearing matching red velvet dresses.

Jennifer and her grandson Dan wearing his favourite wellies in 1993. She was a very proud and active grandmother.

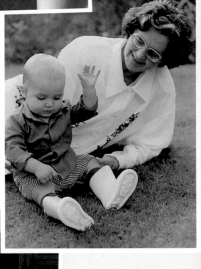

Jennifer stylishly dressed as always, with her granddaughters: Lydia (left) and Eleanor (right) in 1995. Eleanor had just started walking and was very proud. Lydia was preoccupied with her wayward hair, which slides and bobbles struggled to tame.

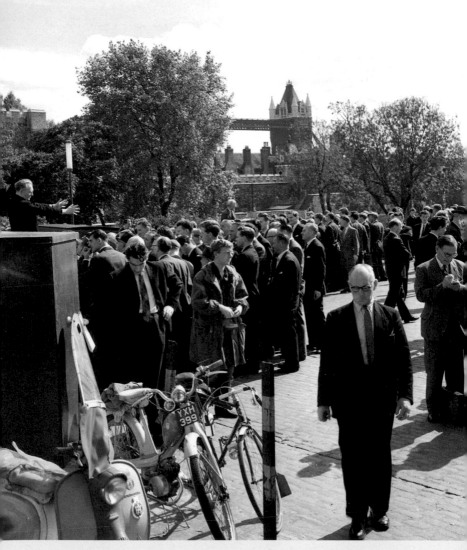

A soapbox speaker at Tower Bridge in the late 1950s, where Fred was a popular entertainer until it came to an abrupt end.

The Millwall Allotments.

Those who have not experienced at first hand
the passions that burn in the hearts of allotment
holders have missed a rare treat in life. Let
a man rent from his local council authority a
pole, or half a pole, or even a mere third of a pole
of of ground for the purpose of growing his vegetables,
and he becomes overnight a Duke, nay a Prince of, the
owner of endless rolling acres of verdant pastures.
Gone forever from his mind are unworthy preoccupations
with the dogs or the Derby, with pubs or parties.
with his pals and pints. More lofty thoughts prevail
these days, thoughts of succulent lettuce in springtime,
ripe tomatoes in autumn, healthy spinach for the
childrens bones, There is nothing he cannot grow in
the winter days, sitting beside his fire thumbing
through Seed catalogues, comparing prices, making
lists and endless notes about rotation and soil
conditions, and fertilises.
Comes the Spring weather, and he is out early
and late, before and after work that is, with his

Page one of the original manuscript of the allotment story, written around
2002. Notice the little bits of sticky paper used to hide mistakes. Also the title:
at some point it changed from Millwall to Mudchute Allotments.

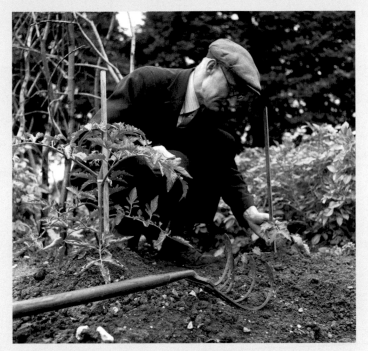

An old man planting seeds in an allotment, around 1950, similar to the Mudchute Allotments where Fred kept his pigs.

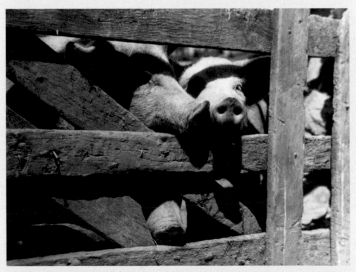

Pigs in a wooden pigsty, similar to the one built by Chip to house Fred's beloved pigs.

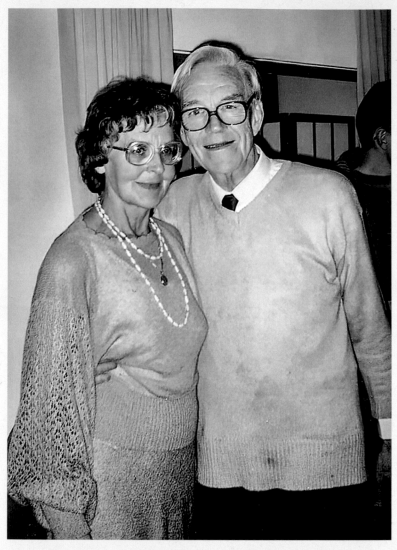

Jennifer and Philip in 2005. Notice my mother is still wearing the same outfit she wore in 1995. My father always wore a shirt and tie, but invariably spoilt the effect with a stained and shapeless old jumper! Bless him.

a bit. I'm more agile than he is. Couldn't I go up the ladder?'

Sister looked at me knowingly.

'I have no doubt that you are more agile. But if you suggested to Fred that he was getting on and was no longer capable of going up a ladder, he would be highly offended. We'll leave it to him.'

Twenty minutes later, Fred came downstairs looking, unusually for him, abashed. The fag that normally hung from his lower lip was not there. He looked different without it.

'What happened, Fred?' we chorused.

Knowing that we were agog with anticipation and that he was the only source of information, just to tease us he took out a battered tobacco tin from his pocket and started rolling another thin fag.

'Oh, Fred. Don't provoke. Tell us what happened.'

He lit his fag, scratched his head and looked at us with his south-west eye, before saying, 'Well, I reckon as 'ow I must be the only bloke in England wot's seen a nun stark naked. I gets up the ladder to the winder, like, an' pokes me 'ead in. "Be off with you, fellow," she calls out. "I gotta ge' in, Sister," I says. "Come back another day, if you must; it's not convenient at the moment." And she splashes water in me face. Well, I wasn't expectin' it, an' I nearly lost me balance. But I grabs the sides of the winder an' hangs on, and says, "I'm sorry, Sister, but I gotta get in. You can't stay in 'ere all night. You'll catch yer death o' cold." Nah, tricky bit is the bath's under the winder, so I 'as ter get in an' over the bath, wiv 'er in it an' not fall in meself.'

'How did you manage that, Fred?'

'Wiv difficulty an' injinuity. Jest bein' smart, like.'

'Fred, you are so clever.'

'Nah, nah, jest smart like,' he said modestly. 'Worse fing was I drops me fag some'ow, an' it floats around the ol' lady. Then I unlocks the door, and Sisters come in, an' now I'm goin' a put me ladders away.'

'Would you like a cup of tea before you go, Fred?'

'Well, now, that's an invitation I can't resist, if you girls will 'ave one wiv me.'

Of course we would. We would like nothing better. So we all sat down in the big kitchen for a cup of tea and some of Mrs B's cake and a good old natter.

Upstairs we heard further sounds of movement and voices, then splashing of water and the gurgling of a waste pipe. Then no more. The Greater Silence had begun.

One memorable Sunday afternoon, Cynthia and I took Sister Monica Joan for a walk. The weather was beautiful, and we decided to take her up to Victoria Park, where there is a lovely lake, and where East Enders would gather with their children in sunny weather. But when the bus arrived it was full, so on the spur of the moment we changed our plan and took the next bus, which was going to Limehouse, and past the canal known as the Cuts. We thought we could have a walk along the towpath. The canal was dug in the nineteenth century to connect the River Lea to the Limehouse Reach of the Thames and was much used by commercial barges until the closure of the docks in the 1970s. It was always a pleasant area for walking.

When we got there, Sister said unexpectedly, 'I don't like the Cuts.'

'Why not, Sister?'

'A grim place. Bad associations.'

'What do you mean?'

'The place of suicides. In the old days, the bad old days, when there was no money, no work for the men, no food for the children, every week a cry would be heard: "Body in the Cuts, body in the Cuts," and always it was a woman. A poor, ragged, half-starved woman, driven to the limits of despair. Once a woman with a baby strapped to her body was dragged out, I was told.'

'Sister, how terrible. Shall we go away?'

'No. I want to go and see it for myself. I haven't been here for forty years, since Beryl died.'

Cynthia and I glanced at each other. We both wanted to hear the story, but didn't want to disturb her thoughts, in case they flitted off on to something quite unconnected and the story was lost. But the dark water, barely moving, seemed to focus her attention, and she continued.

'They told me she jumped off Stinkhouse Bridge one night, and her body was dragged out the next day. I wasn't surprised. No one was. She had a brute of a husband, seven children, another expected, no money, and a hovel to live in – the usual story. It is only surprising more women didn't do it. Every child's fear, you know, was that one day things would get so bad that Mother would jump into the Cuts.'

Sister Monica Joan raised her hand, took hold of the cross that hung around her neck and held it up over the canal. She called out, 'Be sanctified, you black and wicked waters. Rest in peace, Beryl, unloved wife, weeping mother. May the lamentations of your children sanctify these turgid deeps.'

Sister was in good form and continued, 'Do you know what that brute of a husband said when the vicar informed him that his wife was dead, and how she had died?'

'No. What?' we chorused.

'He said, my dears – the vicar himself told us – the husband said, "Spiteful cat. Spiteful to the last. She knows as 'ow today's Newmarket day, and she knows as 'ow I'm a delicate feelin' sort o' chap, so she goes an' kills 'erself jest to put me out of sorts for the races. I knows 'er nasty ways. Spite it was; pure spite." Then he walked out. The vicar was left alone in the derelict kitchen, with seven dirty, hungry children around him, for whom he would have to make some sort of provision, if the father wouldn't. Then the man returned. But he had no thoughts for his children. He walked jauntily up to the vicar, tapped him on the chest and said, "Now you listen 'ere, mate. I won't 'ave no funerals on Friday. That's Epsom day, see? No funerals. I won't 'ave 'er laughin' twice."

'That was the last the vicar saw of him. He didn't turn up for the funeral, which was on a Tuesday, and he simply abandoned his children. All of them ended up in the workhouse.'

Sister Monica Joan said no more, and we continued walking. The sun was pleasant, and the ghosts of the past seemed long since asleep. We came to a wooden seat and sat down. After a few moments enjoying the sun, Sister Monica Joan abruptly stood up.

'The water is not very deep,' she announced, 'I don't see how anyone could drown in it.'

'It is in the middle,' I pointed out. 'It takes cargo barges.'

'But you can see the bottom. Look, you can see the stones.'

'That's only at the edges. Anyway, the water level is low at the moment. I assure you it is deep in the middle.'

'I don't believe it. We shall see.'

Before we could stop her, and she was surprisingly nimble, Sister Monica Joan had crossed the few steps to the canal and now stood ankle-deep at the water's edge.

'There, I told you,' she cried triumphantly, 'the stories about people drowning in the Cuts are just fancy.' And she took another step towards the centre.

'Come back,' screamed Cynthia and I in alarm. We leaped into the water beside her, but Sister was too quick for us.

'Don't be silly,' she called out, taking another step forward. But the Cuts was cut away, and instantly she fell forward into deep water.

Cynthia and I were not the only ones to hurl ourselves in after her. As many as a dozen East Enders dived, fully clothed, into the canal that Sunday afternoon. None of us need have bothered. It was immediately obvious that Sister Monica Joan could swim. Her habit did not absorb the water at once, and it floated around her like the wings of a huge black waterfowl. Her head was held high, and her white veil floated behind her like exotic plumage.

All might have been well, and Sister might have swum back to us, had it not been for the enthusiasm of three local lads who dived in from the other bank. They grabbed hold of her and began swimming back whence they had come.

'No, not that side!' I screamed. 'Come back – this side!' Everyone around, including those in the water, was screaming instructions. We all knew that if the boys landed Sister on the opposite bank there was no towpath exit to the bridge. But the lads did not nor could not understand in all the confusion. They had pulled Sister to the middle of the canal and saw themselves as heroes. A powerful man, with muscles of oak and the speed of an Olympic swimmer, reached them first. He clouted one lad around the ear, pushed the other boy under, took hold of the protesting nun and swam back with her to our side.

Do not ask me how we got Sister Monica Joan back to the convent. The whole process was too complicated and confusing. My memories are hazy: getting her clothes off with modesty and decorum; dozens of wet people offering advice; wondering what on earth to put on her; someone donating a raincoat, a cardigan, a baby's shawl; trying to find her shoes. The swimmer and another man got her to the Commercial Road by giving her a chair-lift. She sat regally on their crossed hands, holding their arms with perfect composure, as though a ducking in the Cuts were a regular experience. Someone must have stopped a lorry in the Commercial Road, because I remember the two men lifting Sister up into the lorry and settling her comfortably. She thanked them with queenly grace, and two tough, strong dockers blushed with pleasure. 'No trouble at all, ma'am,' they said. 'Any time. Good day, ma'am.'

Back at the convent she was put to bed with hot-water

bottles and hot drinks. She slept for twenty-four hours, and when she awoke she appeared to have no memory at all of what had happened. She suffered no ill. It must have been the angels again.

Chapter Fourteen

TAXI!

Sister Monica Joan had a number of relatives whom she decided she must visit. I have described earlier the niece living in Sonning-on-Thames, to whom she bequeathed two fine Chippendale chairs. Another niece and nephew with their three children lived nearer, in Richmond, which was still a tidy distance for a very old lady to travel alone by bus. But, undaunted, she set out.

I am not sure whether she told anyone where she was going (probably not), but once again there was general anxiety in the convent because Sister Monica Joan was missing, it was eight o'clock and time for Compline. No doubt prayers were said for her safety, which must have caught the ear of the Almighty, or whoever oversees these small matters, because at that moment the telephone rang, and the niece in Richmond said that her aunt was with them, enjoying the company of the three children. Asked whether she could stay the night, the niece said it would be difficult, because they had only a small house and there wasn't a spare bed, but her aunt was welcome to sleep on the sofa. At this point Sister Julienne made a tactical error, which she freely admitted later. A night on a sofa would have done Sister Monica Joan no harm whatsoever, but Sister Julienne hesitated and said she really ought to come back to the convent.

Thinking that it was too late in the evening to ask them to put her on a bus, Sister told them to put her in a taxi, which would be paid for on arrival.

It was a grave mistake, which in subsequent days and weeks led to a series of incidents that spun out of control. Sister Monica Joan had probably not been in a London taxicab since they were horse-drawn. As a professed nun she was vowed to a life of poverty, and if she travelled anywhere she took the bus or train, the cheapest available route. A modern taxi was a new and delightful experience.

At lunch the next day, Sister was full of her niece and nephew in Richmond, and their three delightful daughters. 'Such pretty gels, don't you know, so engaging.' She couldn't remember their names, but one of them, poor child, had spots. Such an affliction at that age. She would go that very afternoon to Chrisp Street Market to find a suitable treatment for the one with spots.

She sailed around the market, oblivious to sideways glances and whispered warnings that went before her from the costers, who all kept a wary eye on her since they had been frustrated in their charge of petty theft.

She homed in on a new stall run by a woman with beads and flowers around her neck and in her hair, who sold herb and flower remedies and potions in pretty pots with exotic-sounding names, guaranteed to cure anything. Ingrown toenails, gastric ulcers, piles, failing eyesight, toothache – all could be cured by her remedies. Sister Monica Joan was in a delirium of delight. This was what she had been looking for, all her life, she assured the woman behind the stall – an essence of marigold, a tincture of dog daisy, an infusion of dandelion, and all so simply explained in the little booklet. She pored over the booklet and compared it with her notes on astrology and life forces and earth centres and came to the happy conclusion that all had been revealed. Not only would the one with the spots, sweet child, be cured, but her future would be luminous.

The next day, Sister Julienne had a rather nasty telephone call from the nephew, who said that his aunt had woken the whole house at three o'clock in the morning with a garbled story about flower essence, and if you have a bad toe rub it on your toe and it will get better, and if you have a tummy ache rub it on your tummy and the ache will go away, and if the one with the spots rubs it on her spots they will go away, and wasn't it wonderful? The nephew had replied that it was not at all wonderful. He and his wife had to go to work the next day, and the children had to go to school, and did she realise what time of the night it was? Sister Monica Joan had replied that yes, she thought she knew, but she was so sure the one with the spots ought to hear the good news straight away, so could she speak to her? The nephew had replied certainly not, it was ten past three, and the girl had to go to school. She was doing her O levels and needed her sleep.

Sister Julienne was apologising and saying that she had no idea Sister Monica Joan was active in the middle of the night, when the nephew interrupted to say that that was not the end of the story by any means. About an hour later they were all woken again, and Sister Monica Joan explained that she didn't want the one with the spots to think she was being specially favoured, but spots were such an affliction at that age, didn't he know, nor did she want the two younger gels to feel left out, so she had a little present for them also, which she would give to them personally.

After that, the nephew said, he had disconnected the telephone, and Sister Julienne agreed that under the circumstances it was the best thing he could have done.

The following Saturday, Sister Monica Joan decided to go to Richmond again. She discussed it fully with everyone around the big dining table. She must be sure to see those dear gels again, and how exciting to discover you have young and pretty great-nieces that you didn't know you had, and it reminded her of her own young days with her sisters in the big house and all the fun they used to have.

Sister Julienne was glad to know at least where she was going on this occasion, and telephoned the nephew to tell him to expect his aunt. She made quite sure that Sister Monica Joan had enough money for the bus fare.

But a humble London double-decker was not part of Sister Monica Joan's plans. Having once experienced the delights of a London taxicab, buses were out of the question. Oh, the pleasure and the grandeur of sitting alone in the spacious interior while a competent driver weaves his way through the streets. None of the awful business of having to get off one bus and wait anxiously for another. No standing around – just go straight from Poplar to Richmond (about fifteen miles through Central London). Sister Monica Joan was delighted with her new-found ease of transport. No fussing, looking for your bus pass. No fumbling for pennies and shillings to pay the bus conductor. And it didn't seem to cost anything. You just had to say, 'Payment will be met on arrival,' and off he went, dear man.

The nephew did not complain the first two times he was expected to finance the taxi fare, but, after the third occasion, he put through a gentle phone call to Sister Julienne asking her, as tactfully as he could, if she could provide his aunt with sufficient money to pay for her own taxi. Sister, who, with mounting alarm at the depletion of the convent's petty cash, had paid for four return taxis, agreed that things were getting out of hand and that she would have to do something, although she was not sure what. The nephew was particular to say that they were all delighted with his aunt's visits, and the girls adored her and would sit listening to her for hours. She was enchanting. It was just the taxi fares . . .

There was considerable discussion amongst the nuns as to how best to control the mounting problem. Sister Julienne had a very serious discussion with Sister Monica Joan about the vows of poverty, the need to economise for the sake of running the convent, the expense of taxi fares, and the need to take the bus wherever possible. Sister Monica Joan was very amenable and fully understood that she had been extravagant, so she agreed to take the bus in future. But perhaps she forgot. Or perhaps she could not resist the temptation when she saw a shiny black taxicab in the street. Or perhaps her intentions were good, but it was raining, and Sister Monica Joan could not abide the rain. Whatever the reason, the situation continued as before. Sister Julienne felt obliged to refund to the nephew all the taxi fares incurred to date, because a nun is the responsibility of the convent, and not of her family.

The Sisters had further discussions. At the start of her next journey, Novice Ruth took Sister Monica Joan to the bus stop, put her on the correct bus, paid the bus conductor, and told him where she was to get off. But Sister Monica Joan was crafty, and she always got what she wanted. She thanked Novice Ruth kindly for her assistance, sweetly waved goodbye and quite simply got off at the next stop and took a taxi.

Things were going too far. Sister Julienne was obliged to inform the Reverend Mother Jesu Emanuel. Large sums of money were regularly leaking out of the convent funds, and she could not seem to control it. A Chapter meeting of all the Sisters at the Mother House in Chichester was convened, and the financial adviser was requested to be present. Thirty-two Sisters who worked in the Mother House attended, and many of them were very critical of Sister Monica Joan. Her behaviour was outrageous. She had first brought scandal to the Order through a court case for alleged theft, and now, instead of being humble and contrite as any other nun would be, she was spending money with reckless abandon. Why should they have to skimp and save and live a life of poverty while she was riding around London like a duchess?

The Reverend Mother pointed out to the younger Sisters that Sister Monica Joan had given over fifty years of dedicated service to the poorest of the poor, in conditions of unimaginable squalor, and it was the policy of the Order to allow privileges and comforts to elderly Sisters who had retired from nursing. Two or three of the elderly Sisters spoke up to say that they had also given lives of dedicated service to the poor and needy, and that they defined 'comforts and privileges' as jam on Sundays, or an occasional cup of tea in bed. They could not approve of taxis all over the place. It was a question of what was reasonable.

The Reverend Mother sighed; Sister Monica Joan had never been reasonable. She asked the financial adviser, an independent auditor and accountant, for his opinion.

The accountant said that he had carefully studied the finances of the Order, and had observed that Sister Monica Joan's dowry to the Order in 1906, when she made her life vows, was greater than that of all the other Sisters put together. In addition, a very large inheritance, which she had received in 1922 on the death of her mother, had immediately gone into the convent funds. Had it not been for these two large deposits of money, the accountant questioned whether the Sisters would have been able to continue their work at all.

That settled it. The Chapter ruled that finances should be made available to Sister Julienne to use at her discretion. There were still a few sour faces and mutters of 'not fair', which the Reverend Mother dispelled by saying that she was sure that all the Sisters would be relieved by the decision, as many would be anxious at the thought of an old lady roaming alone around London by bus – especially as her mind was wandering, as had been made clear by the recent scandal. 'Let's face it. She's senile and shouldn't be let out,' muttered one of the younger Sisters. To this the Reverend Mother replied sharply that the remark was uncharitable, and she would not countenance the thought of Sister Monica Joan being confined to the House like a prisoner.

Sister Julienne was relieved by the decision of the Chapter and was able to finance several more taxi fares to and from Richmond with no further anxiety. Nonetheless, she had another little talk with Sister Monica Joan about limiting the number of visits, the need for economy and the vows of poverty. Sister Monica Joan must have taken this to heart; perhaps her conscience had been pricked by the reminder of her life vows, or perhaps she just wanted a bit of diversion. After all, she had always been an adventurous soul, seeking out a challenge.

The next thing we heard was that she had been seen by many witnesses standing at the traffic lights by the Blackwall Tunnel. When the lights turned red and the traffic stopped, she would totter into the road, round the front of the cars and lorries, tap on the window of a car, and ask the astonished driver to take her to Richmond.

Whatever might be said of nuns, thumbing lifts from strange men is not the way they are expected to behave. The reaction of the drivers can only be imagined. Sister Monica Joan would have been wearing the full monastic habit of her Order. If you were a businessman going to your next appointment, such an apparition weaving its way unsteadily into the road must have looked like a visitation from God – or perhaps the devil. When the apparition tapped on your window and started a long, convoluted yarn about pretty nieces in Richmond, and how she had got a new lotion from the woman in the market for the one with spots, but she suspected blackheads really, guaranteed to make them go away, and that was why she needed to get to Richmond, but buses were so difficult, you would probably have thought you were going a bit mad, particularly if the business lunch had been of the liquid variety.

Without exception, the drivers refused, but Sister Monica Joan persisted in what to her mind was a perfectly reasonable request. The man had a car, and she did not, she would point out. It would surely be no inconvenience to him to make a small detour to Richmond? She knew the address – what was the difficulty? She was a lady inclined to become extremely cross and snappish if she did not get her own way, and many of the conversations ended in acrimony.

Several times, while she was still talking, the lights turned green, and the traffic started up again. Lorries in the free-moving lane passed alarmingly close as she stood in the road. The car driver, who would still be trying to reason with her, could not start, and there would be honking and hooting and shouts from frustrated motorists piled up behind. Eventually (and this happened several times), she would accept that the car driver was not going to Richmond and would not divert his journey to take her, and she would totter back to the pavement, only to try again when the lights turned red and another car stopped on the nearside lane.

After half a dozen such attempts, she was caught in the act by two policemen, who observed her actions for a few minutes and then apprehended her for causing an obstruction to the traffic and for endangering her life and that of others. Sister Monica Joan was very sensitive about policemen and protested violently at finding herself between two of them, and being escorted back to the convent.

After this little escapade, Sister Julienne begged her to take taxis, and hang the expense.

A printed letter arrived for Sister Monica Joan from Wandsworth Borough Council, stating that a lady's handbag containing a little money, a prayer book, a pair of spectacles and a set of false teeth had been found and awaited her collection at a lost property office in West London. Sister Julienne was taking no chances. A taxi was ordered to collect Sister Monica Joan, to take her to the address on the letter and to return her to the convent.

Four hours later the taxi returned. The driver said that when he reached West London, she said that she had forgotten or lost the piece of paper giving the address. She knew she should be going to a lost property office but she was not sure which one. So she had instructed him to drive to all the lost property offices in the area, which amounted to fifteen throughout Fulham, Putney, Chelsea, Wimbledon, Kingston, Twickenham and as far west as Hampton Court. No handbag was reclaimed. He must have missed the one where it was, he said. Anyway, the old lady seemed to have enjoyed herself. She'd had a nice day out. She had enjoyed going over Hammersmith Bridge so much that she had instructed him to go back, and then to go over it again, he said. He had looked after her and brought her home safely. The cost was so astronomical that Sister Julienne thought she would have to consult the Reverend Mother again. Where would it all end?

Novice Ruth was the first person up that morning. She was approaching her first-year professional vows and wanted an hour of private devotion alone in the chapel before her Sisters joined her. The time was 4 a.m., and, it being summer, the dawn was breaking and light was returning to the world. She walked quietly along the passage, turned the corner and found Sister Monica Joan lying on the floor. She was breathing, but her eyes were wide open and staring, her pulse was bounding and she was twitching intermittently. She had wet herself and could not be roused. Novice Ruth fetched a pillow and placed it under her head and wrapped a warm blanket around her. Then she telephoned the doctor and woke Sister Julienne. Together they carried the unconscious figure back to her room and laid her on the bed. Twenty minutes later the doctor arrived, examined the patient and confirmed what they had both suspected: Sister Monica Joan had had a stroke. She did not regain consciousness and died that evening, at the hour of Compline. The last words of the last office of the day are: 'Lord, grant us a quiet night and a perfect end.'

Peace at the hour of death is one of the greatest blessings that God can give. Death can be very terrible, but peace can transform it. Sister Monica Joan received no intrusive medical treatment, no drugs, no investigations into the cause of the stroke, no attempts to prolong her life or to delay her death. She received loving nursing care from her Sisters and was able to die in peace. This is the perfect end.

Her body lay at rest for two days in the convent chapel, and local people came to pay their respects. Then she was taken to the Mother House in Chichester for the funeral service.

The death of Sister Monica Joan affected me deeply. I had not expected her to die; I had somehow believed that she was indestructible. I could not reconcile myself to the loss. The magic and mystery of that extraordinary woman haunted me. Suddenly, all the beauty and fun and bewitchment that she encapsulated was gone, leaving me utterly bereft.

Aware of my state of mind, Sister Julienne said to me one day, with her usual twinkle, 'I was thinking about Sister Monica Joan this morning in chapel. Perhaps it was rather naughty of me, but the Old Testament reading about Elijah going up to Heaven in a fiery chariot prompted the thought: don't you think perhaps that Sister Monica Joan went straight to Heaven by taxi?'

PART VI
FRED

In which Fred acquires a pig

Remember the end of the first chapter simply entitled 'Fred'? My mother finishes with a single line: 'But Fred's triumph was yet to come.' Well, this chapter, also from *Call the Midwife*, concerns that triumph. It is another of the stories we liked to read when giving our talks and, as was customary, my father took the part of Fred. When he got to the line, '*Wha' we needs is a red-hot poker to stick up his arse, like wha' they do with camels in the desert . . .*' he had our audiences in fits of laughter, and as with 'Sister Monica Joan gets stuck in the bath', it took several moments before we could resume the reading.

Sister Julienne, Sister in charge at Nonnatus House, features significantly in this chapter. It ends with all the nuns assembling for evening prayers; inspired writing, and I think some of my mother's best.

Chapter Fifteen

THE BOTTOM DROPPED OUT OF PIGS

Always expect the unexpected, and you will never go wrong. Fred had suffered a severe setback from the enforced closure of his quail and toffee-apple empire, and was looking round for something new. The unexpected came from a chance remark Mrs B made as she bustled into the kitchen muttering, 'I don' know what fings is comin' to. The price o' bacon these days! I've never seen nuffink like it.'

Fred slapped his shovel down on the floor, raising a cloud of ash, and shouted: 'Pigs! That's the answer. Pigs. They was doin' it in the war, an' it can be done again.'

Mrs B rushed over to him, broom in hand. 'You messy bugger, messin' up my kitchen.'

She held the broom aggressively, ready to strike. But Fred neither heard nor saw. He grabbed her round the waist and twirled her round and round in a frenzied dance.

'You got it, old girl, you 'as. Why didn't I think on it? Pigs.'

He made snorting, honking noises, supposed to represent a pig, which did not improve his looks at all. Mrs B extricated herself from his embrace, and poked him in the chest with the broom handle.

'You crazy—' she started shouting, and he yelled back. When two Cockneys are engaged in a shouting match, it is impossible to understand the lingo.

Breakfast was over, and we heard the Sisters' footsteps. They appeared in the doorway, and the slanging match stopped. In high excitement, Fred explained that he had just had a brilliant idea. He would keep a pig. It could live in the chicken run, which he could easily convert into a pigsty, and in no time at all the pig would be ready for the bacon factory, and his fortune would be made.

Sister Julienne was enchanted. She loved pigs. She had been brought up on a farm, and knew a lot about them. She said that Fred could have all the peelings and waste from Nonnatus House, and advised him to go round the local cafés begging similar favours. Shyly she asked if she might come to see the pig when it was installed in the hen/pig house.

Fred wasn't one to hang around. Within a matter of days, the pigsty was complete. He and his daughter Dolly pooled their resources and a pink, squealing little creature was soon purchased.

Sister Julienne was profuse in her praise.

'You've got a fine pig, there, Fred. A real beauty. You can tell by the width of the shoulders. You've made a good choice.'

She gave him one of her sparkling smiles and Fred turned as pink as the pig.

Fred yielded to Sister Julienne for advice about bran mash and nut mix, as well as supplies of food waste from local cafés and greengrocers. They were frequently seen in deep and earnest conversation, Fred sucking his tooth and whistling inwardly as he concentrated on the detail. Sister also advised him on hay and water and mucking out, and she impressed us all with her knowledge in the art of pig rearing.

It was a busy and happy time for Fred. Each day at breakfast we heard details of the pig's progress, her lusty appetite and rapid growth. As the weeks passed, mucking out consumed more of Fred's time and labour. However, this proved to be a moneymaker. Most small houses had tiny back gardens, no more than a yard in most cases, but quite sufficient to grow a few things. Tomatoes were popular, and so, surprisingly, were grapevines, which grew exceedingly well in Poplar and produced succulent fruit. Word soon got round, and Fred's pig shit was in great demand. He concluded that there was no losing with pigs. The more he fed her, the more thick, black stuff she excreted, and the more money he made. Within a few weeks the sale of manure had covered the initial cost of the piglet.

The whole of Nonnatus House, Sisters and lay staff alike, took a deep interest in the pig and Fred's financial aspirations. We read in the papers that the price of meat was rising, and concluded that Fred had been very shrewd.

However, the vagaries and vicissitudes of the market are notorious. Demand fell. The bottom dropped out of pigs.

The blow was heavy. Fred was glum. All that feeding and mucking and raking. All the plans and hopes. And now the pig was hardly worth the cost of slaughter. No wonder the bounce had gone out of Fred's bent little legs. No wonder his north-east eye drooped.

Sunday was a day of rest in Nonnatus House. After church we were all gathered in the kitchen, having coffee and cakes left by Mrs B from her Saturday bake. Fred was packing up to leave, but Sister Julienne invited him to join us at the big table. Conversation turned to the pig; his fag drooped.

'What'm I goin' to do wiv 'er? She's costin' me money to feed an' I can't ge' nuffink for 'er.'

Everyone sympathised and muttered 'hard luck' and 'shame', but Sister Julienne was silent. She stared at him intently, and then said, clearly and positively, 'Breed from her, Fred. You could keep her as a breeding sow. There will always be a market for good healthy piglets, and when prices pick up, as they will, you could get a good price for them. And don't forget, a sow always delivers between twelve and eighteen piglets.'

Such advice – so obvious, so simple, yet so unexpected! Fred's mouth fell open, and his fag dropped on to the table.

Picking it up with an apology, he stubbed it out in the ashtray. Unfortunately it was not an ashtray; it was Sister Evangelina's meringue, which she had been on the point of eating. She remonstrated with characteristic vigour.

Fred was abashed and apologetic. He picked up the meringue, brushed off the ash, picked the fag end out of the cream and handed it back to Sister Evangelina. 'Piglets. Tha's the answer. I'll be a pig breeder. I'll be the best pig breeder on the Isle.'

Sister Evangelina snorted, and pushed the meringue away from her with disgust. But Fred noticed none of this. He was in a trance, muttering, 'Piglets, piglets, I'll breed pigs, that's what I'll do, I will.'

Sister Julienne, practical and tactful, handed another meringue to Sister Evangelina, and said, 'You will have to take the *Pig Breeders' Guide*, Fred, and find a good stud boar. I can help you, if you need help in the first instance. My brother is a farmer so I can ask him to send a copy.'

And that was how it all started. The *Pig Breeders' Guide* arrived, and Fred and Sister Julienne were soon poring over it. It was disconcerting to see Fred attempting to read, because he had to hold the page to the left of his south-west eye in order to read anything at all. Even when he could make out a sentence or two, the language of pig breeders was completely foreign to him, and he could not have managed without Sister Julienne, who translated the strange jargon into comprehensible Cockney.

A good stud boar was selected, a telephone call made, an agreement reached, and a small open truck arrived from Essex.

Sister Julienne could hardly contain her excitement. Instructing Sister Bernadette to take charge of the House in her absence, she put on her outdoor veil and cloak, pulled a bicycle out of the shed, and cycled off to Fred's house.

*

The Essex farmer was a rural gentleman of settled habits. His thoughts, as he drove his open truck with his stud boar into the heart of London's Docklands, have not been revealed to us. The boar, resting his head contentedly on the side of the truck, jogged along for several miles without arousing much interest, but once in the more densely populated streets of London it was a different story. All the way through Dagenham, Barking, East Ham, West Ham and down to Cubitt Town on the Isle of Dogs, the pig drew crowds. He was a large animal whose only exercise was that of copulation. His nature was comparatively docile, but in ten years his tusks had never been cut, and in consequence he looked more ferocious than he really was.

As the truck turned in at the end of the street, Sister Julienne arrived on her bicycle and met Fred. Together they approached the farmer, who stared at them without saying a word. Sister Julienne stood on tiptoe, looking over the edge of the truck, and brushed back her veil, which had been blowing towards the pig's tusks.

'Oh, he's a beautiful fellow,' she whispered excitedly.

The farmer looked at her, sucked his pipe, and said, 'I don't believe this.'

He asked to see the sow. The entry to Fred's yard was via a side passage that ran between the houses, at the end of which was the boundary wall to the docks. The Thames ran behind it. The farmer was thus confronted with the towering sides of ocean-going cargo vessels.

'They're never going to believe this. Never,' he muttered, as he stooped to pick up his pipe and the keys that had fallen from his hands.

He was directed into Fred's yard.

'There she is, an' lookin' for a bi' of fun from that there big bugger o' your'n.'

'Fun!' growled the farmer. 'This bit of fun will cost you one pound, cash in hand.'

Fred knew the cost, and had the money ready, but grumbled nonetheless. 'Cor – pound a poke – that's more'n they gets up West, that is.'

Sister Julienne remonstrated: 'It's no good grumbling, Fred. A pound is the going rate, so you had better pay up.'

The farmer eyed the nun strangely, but Fred handed over the money without another word.

The farmer pocketed the cash and said, 'Right! We'll bring him round.'

But that was easier said than done.

A crowd had gathered, and was growing all the time – word travels fast on the Isle. The farmer backed his truck up against the passage, lowered the rear trailer board, and leaped into the truck to drive the boar down, but the boar refused to budge. A pig's eyesight is poor, and, to a creature accustomed to the open countryside of Essex, the passage must have looked like the black hole into hell.

'Get up and help me,' shouted the farmer to Fred.

Together they pushed and walloped and shouted at the boar, which got nasty, and looked as if it might be tempted to use its tusks after all. The crowd in the street gasped, and mothers pulled their children back as the boar, slowly and tentatively, descended the ramp on its tiny trotters and entered the passage. Even then it was not plain sailing. The alley was narrow, and the boar very nearly got stuck. The two men pushed from behind. Sister Julienne ran through the house, through the pig yard and the outside gate, and into the passage with turnip tops in her hand, which she said would entice the pig forward. She held them under its nose, but still it would not move.

Fred had an idea. 'Wha' we needs is a red-hot poker to stick up his arse, like wha' they do with camels in the desert when they wants 'em to go over a bridge. Camels won' go over water, you know.'

'You stick a red-hot poker up his arse, and I'll stick one up yours, mate,' the farmer threatened, and continued pushing.

Eventually the boar was coaxed down the passage into Fred's yard. A crowd of children followed, and more went into neighbouring gardens and hung over the fence.

The farmer got cross. He spoke with slow emphasis.

'You'll have to clear this crowd away. Pigs are shy animals; they won't perform in front of an audience.'

Again, Sister Julienne took charge. She spoke with quiet authority to the children, and they crept away. She, Fred and the farmer went into the house and shut the door. But Sister could not resist the temptation to peep out through the curtains to see how the sow took to her 'husband', as she insisted on calling the boar.

'Oh, Fred, I don't think she likes him – look, she's pushing him away. He's definitely interested, do you see?'

Fred stood by the window, sucking his tooth.

'No, no, not like that!' cried Sister Julienne, wringing her hands in anguish. 'You mustn't bite him. That's not the way. Now she's running. Fred, I'm afraid she might not accept him. What do you think?'

Fred didn't know what to think.

'That's better. There's a good girl. She's getting more interested, do you see, Fred? Isn't it wonderful?'

Fred grew alarmed.

'He'll kill 'er, he will. Look at 'im, the big bugger. He's biting her. Look 'ere, I'm not standin' fer this, not no 'ow. He'll kill 'er, he will, or break 'er legs or somefink. I'm gonna put a stop to this, I am. It's barbaric, I tells yer.'

Sister had to restrain him

'It's all perfectly natural. That's the way they do it, Fred.'

Fred was not easily pacified. Sister and the farmer had to hold him back until it was all over.

The nuns were assembled in the chapel, kneeling in private prayer. The bell for Vespers sounded just as Sister Julienne entered Nonnatus House. Flushed and excited, she raced along the corridor, leaving behind footsteps of a sticky and highly pungent substance on the tiled floor. In haste, she composed herself; took her place at the lectern, and read:

'Sisters, be sober, be vigilant, for your adversary the devil roareth around like a raging lion, seeking whom he may devour.'

One or two of the Sisters looked up from their prayers and glanced sideways at her. A few sniffed suspiciously.

She continued:

'Thine adversary roareth in the midst of thy congregation. Thine enemy hath defiled thy holy place.'

The sniffs got louder, and the Sisters glanced at each other.

'But as for me, I walk with the godly.'

The sacristan filled the censer with an unusually large quantity of incense and swung it vigorously.

'In my prosperity I said I shall never be cast down—' smoke filled the air '—but thou, oh Lord, hath seen my pride and sent my misfortune to humble me.'

There was unrest amongst the Sisters. Those kneeling closest to Sister Julienne shuffled a little distance from her. It cannot be easy to shuffle sideways whilst on your knees and wearing monastic habit, but in extremis it can be managed.

'But thou dost turn thy face from me, and I was troubled, and I gat me to my Lord, right humbly.'

The incense swung furiously, smoke billowing out.

'And I will say unto my Lord, I am unclean. I am unfit to dwell in Thy Holy Place.'

Coughing broke out.

'And I cried aloud, What profit is there in me? I am undone. I shall go down into the Pit. Oh Lord, hear my prayer. Let my cry come unto Thee.'

Eventually, and not before time, Vespers concluded. The Sisters, red-eyed, choking and spluttering, filed out of the chapel.

It took a long time for Sister Julienne to live down the opprobrium of having filled the chapel with the odour of pig shit, and I am sure that God forgave her long before her Sisters.

PART VII

CHUMMY

In which Chummy meets her man

These two chapters, taken from *Farewell to the East End*, follow on from 'The Captain's Daughter' and conclude Chummy's story. Chummy, tongue-tied and awkward in the presence of the opposite sex, finally meets her man. I particularly love the scene where the girls are getting ready for the wedding; I can just imagine the flurry of excitement. The writing is full of warmth and humour and, by the end, we feel as if Chummy has become a friend and we are sorry to see her go.

Chapter Sixteen

ON THE SHELF

A knock at the door. Sister Monica Joan was in the hallway. I was just coming downstairs. She opened the door, then banged it shut and started to draw the bolts across. I went up to her.

'Sister, what's the matter?'

She did not answer coherently, but muttered and clucked to herself as she fumbled with the bolts; but they were large and heavy, and her bony fingers had not the strength with which to draw them.

'See here, child, pull this one, pull it hard. We must firm up the battlements, lower the portcullis.'

Another knock at the door.

'But Sister, dear, there's someone at the door. We can't keep them out. It might be important.'

She continued fussing.

'Oh, drat this thing! Why won't you help me?'

'I'm going to open the door, Sister. We can't keep people out. There might be someone in labour.'

I opened the door. A policeman stood there. But Sister was in readiness. She had her crucifix in her hand and held it forward with an outspread arm, thrusting it in his face.

'Stand back, stand back, I adjure you. In the name of Christ, retreat!'

Her voice was quavering with passion, and her poor old arm was trembling, so that the crucifix was rocking and shaking a few inches from his nose.

'You shall not enter. You see before you a Soldier of Christ, girt with the Armour of Salvation, 'gainst which the Jaws of Hell shall not prevail.'

The policeman's face was a study. I tried to intervene.

'But Sister, dear, it's not—'

'Get thee behind me, Satan. Like Horatio I stand alone on the bridge to face the Midian hordes. Lay down thy sword. Desist, thou Scourge of Israel.'

With that she shut the door, then turned to me and gave me one of her naughty winks.

'That will see them off. They won't try again.'

Poor Sister. I understood her aversion to policemen, and sympathised. But perhaps the policeman had called about something to do with our work. It would not have been the first time that a bobby on the beat had been asked to 'go an' call the midwife, deary. I reckons I'm in labour.'

'I'll go and see what he wants. But I won't let him in. I promise you, Sister.'

I opened the door a few inches and slipped out. Sister Monica Joan banged it shut behind me, nearly catching my ankle.

The policeman was standing in the street, looking as though he did not quite know what to do next. A bicycle was propped against the railings.

'You must excuse her. She does not like . . .'

Then I recognised him. It was the copper whom Chummy had knocked over when she was learning to ride her bicycle and who had also accompanied the police sergeant in his investigations about the stolen jewellery. I burst out laughing.

'Oh, it's you. We seem to meet a lot. What do you want this time?'

'I'm not here on police business; you can tell Sister and calm her fears. I've brought a bicycle back, that is all. I told the nurse I would.'

'Which nurse?'

'I don't know her name. The very tall one.'

'Chummy. What are you doing with her bike?'

'I sent her back by taxi, because I did not think she was in a fit condition to ride.'

'What?' I exclaimed, thinking he meant that she was drunk. 'When?'

'This morning at about six o'clock.'

'Good God! Where did you find her?'

'In the docks.'

'In the docks! Drunk and incapable in the docks, at six o'clock in the morning! My God! This is a side of Chummy we knew nothing about. She's a dark horse. You wait till I tell the girls. Was it a wild party, or something?'

He was smiling. He was an interesting-looking man who was probably younger than he appeared. He had an ugly-attractive sort of face, and a scar ran up the side of his cheek almost to the cheekbone. This might have made him look grim, but as he smiled his dark eyes danced with humour.

'No. It was no party, and she was not drunk. I am not sure of the details, but apparently a baby was born on one of the ships, and your nurse Chummy went to deliver it.'

I knew nothing about the drama of the night and stared at him in amazement.

'I saw the nurse staggering along the quayside as my colleague and I were talking with the nightwatchman. It had been a stormy night, and he said that she had climbed up the rope ladder. So presumably she had to climb down again. When I saw her, she looked as if she were on the verge of collapse. She hardly knew where she was going. So I told her not to ride the bike and ordered a taxi. I am now returning the bike,' he added more formally, 'and would like you to sign for it.'

I signed, and he thanked me and turned to go. But then he hesitated and half turned back.

'I was wondering . . .' And then he stopped. Silence.

'Yes? Wondering what?'

'Oh, just thinking . . .' Another silence.

'Well, unless I know what you are thinking, I can't help you, can I?'

'No, of course not.' More silence. 'How is she?'

'Who? Chummy?'

'Yes.'

'Well, I don't know. I didn't know there was anything wrong with her.'

'I'm not sure. I hope not. She looked all in when I saw her, and . . .' His voice trailed off.

'Oh, that's nothing, I assure you. We are frequently "all in". Sometimes the work gets very heavy, and we are often out for long hours. It can be quite exhausting, sometimes. But we get over it. Chummy will, you'll see.'

'I hope so.' Another long silence, in which he looked as if he wanted to say more. I waited.

'Look, tell her I brought back the bike . . .' He stopped again. 'I felt responsible for her in a way this morning, when I saw her staggering along the quayside. She hardly knew where she was going and would have killed herself on a bike in the East India Dock Road. I suppose I just wanted to reassure myself that she is all right now.'

'Well, I honestly don't know. And if you will excuse me, I have to go. I have the morning visits to make, and it's getting late. If you want to know how she is, you had better come back later.' He nodded. 'But come back when you are not on duty, and not in uniform. You might meet Sister Monica Joan again!'

A few days later we were relaxing in our sitting room. The pressure of work had subsided. Then there was a knock at the door. Trixie groaned.

'Here comes trouble. Someone in labour. Who's on call?'

She came back a few minutes later with a wicked grin on her face.

'There's a young man to see you, Chummy.'

'Oh whoopee! It must be my brother, Wizard Prang! He's on leave from the RAF. Pilot, you know. Commissioned officer and all that. Don't know what he does, actually, now that the war is over, but he seems to enjoy it. Ask him to come up, old girl. Not too fast. We'd better tidy up, eh, girls?'

Cynthia, Chummy and I set about clearing away the dirty mugs, plates, papers, magazines, shoes and bits of uniform that were lying around the place. If Chummy's brother, Wizard Prang, was anything like his sister, and from the name it sounded as if he would be, this was going to be a rare treat.

A tall man entered the room. I recognised him at once as the policeman, in plain clothes. Chummy, who couldn't handle men, instantly went bright red and started spluttering. Trixie, who always liked to stir things up, said innocently, 'This is PC David Thompson, and he wants to see you, Chummy.'

'Oh, Great Scott! Me? There must be some mistake. It can't be me.'

She swallowed hard, and her arm jerked sideways, knocking over a table lamp, which fell on to the record player, where our favourite 78 was spinning round. There was a ghastly screeching sound as the needle dragged across the record.

'Oh, clumsy clot! Oh silly me! Now what have I done?' Chummy's voice was distressed.

'You've ruined the Eartha Kitt, that's what you've done, you chump.' Trixie sounded cross. 'That was "Easy Does It", something *you* need to learn to do, you idiot.'

'Oh, sorry, girls. Frightfully sorry and all that. I know I'm a liability. Here, I'll stop the dratted thing.'

Chummy moved, and there was another crash as she knocked over a table of coffee mugs.

'Lawks! What next?' was her anguished cry.

There was a guffaw of masculine laughter.

'David is the policeman you knocked over last year,' said Trixie wickedly. 'He wants to see you.'

'Oh, crikey! Not that again! I didn't mean . . .'

Chummy's voice trailed away into nothingness. Her embarrassment was all-consuming. David looked abashed, in the presence of four girls and a chaotic situation that somehow – he did not know how – he seemed to have provoked. Cynthia came to the rescue, her low voice easing the tension. She picked up the coffee mugs and scooped up the instant coffee from the carpet.

'Nonsense. Of course David hasn't come about last year's accident. Would you like a cup of coffee? There may be some bits of fluff in it, but you can pick them off when they float to the top.' With a few words she put everyone at their ease. 'We were talking about Chummy's extraordinary adventure in the docks the other night.'

'That is why I came.' He turned to Chummy. 'It was a very brave thing you did. Are you all right now?'

'Lawks, yes. Nothing wrong with me. Bounce up like a cork, I do. But how did you know about it, actually?'

'I was there. I saw you coming along the quayside. Don't you remember?'

'No.' Chummy looked vague.

'Well, I do. I think I will always remember the way you looked when you got off that boat. You deserve a medal.'

'Me? Why?'

'For all that you did that night.'

'Oh, fiddlesticks. That was nothing. Anyone would have done the same.'

'I do not think so. I really don't.'

Chummy could not be induced to say anything more. She sat on the edge of her chair, stiff and awkward, looking as though she wished herself a thousand miles away.

The evening passed pleasantly. Policemen and nurses always have a lot in common. I had found from previous experience, living in nurses' homes, that if we wanted to throw an impromptu party, we only had to send an invitation round to the nearest police station and we would be flooded with healthy young coppers, eager to try their chances. David certainly enjoyed himself, being the centre of the attention among four young girls, even though one of them was too shy to talk.

Inevitably, the conversation turned to Chummy's experience in the docks, and in particular to the ship's woman, who held a morbid fascination for us. We were agog to hear more about the life of such a woman and tried to get Chummy to talk about her. But it was no use. Poor Chummy might have been able to be expansive with us girls, but in mixed company she was speechless with discomfort. In those days, it must be remembered, even amongst midwives who saw just about everything, sexual matters were either unmentionable, or referred to obliquely and with exaggerated delicacy. And the life of a ship's woman was in no way delicate!

We asked David if he had heard of such a character. He assured us that, although every crew might wish to have one, a ship's woman was pretty rare, because of the strict controls on trading vessels. 'But they do exist, as you have found out.' He looked sideways at Chummy with an amused grin. She persisted in looking at the carpet, biting her lips and chewing her fingernails.

The clock struck eleven. David stood up to leave. Cynthia said, 'This has been so nice. We do hope you will come again. Chummy, would you show David out, while we tidy up?'

Chummy reluctantly stood up and cast an appealing glance at Cynthia, who refused to notice her distress. In silence they left the room, and a few minutes later we heard the front door close.

Chummy reappeared, looking pink, giggly and bewildered.

'Well?' we all said in chorus.

'He has asked me to go out with him.'

'Of course. What did you expect?'

'Nothing.'

'Nothing?'

'No.'

'Well, why do you think he came here, all dressed up in his best suit with a clean shirt and a new tie?'

'Was he? I didn't notice.'

'Of course he was. Anyone could see that.'

'But why? I don't understand.'

'Because he likes you. That's why.'

'He can't do. Not in that way, anyway. I'm not pretty. I'm not even attractive. I'm too big, and I'm clumsy and awkward. My feet are too big. I fall over things. I never know what to say to anyone. My mater can't take me anywhere; she says I'm on the shelf.'

'Well, your mater is an ass.'

His first visit left the convent in a flurry of excitement. Even the Sisters were twittering with interest. It was the last thing anyone had expected. The evening of Chummy's first date was the occasion for unsolicited advice and useless assistance. First, what should she wear? She produced a few clothes from her wardrobe, none of them very attractive.

'You must have something new.'

'But what?'

We all borrowed and swapped each other's clothes, but nothing that we wore fitted Chummy, so in the end we sighed hopelessly and loaned her a pretty scarf. She was also in a dither over what she should talk about.

'I'm no good with boys. I have never been dated by a boy before. What am I going to say?'

'Look, don't be daft. He's not a boy, he's a grown man, and

he wouldn't have asked you out if he hadn't any reason to think you are interesting.'

'Oh, lawks! This is going to be a disaster, I know it. What if I fall over, or say something bally silly? My mater says you can't take me anywhere.'

'Well, your mater's not taking you out, is she? Forget "Mater". Think of David.'

The doorbell rang, and Chummy fell over the doormat, crashing into the door.

'Enjoy yourself,' we all whispered in chorus, but she didn't look as though she would.

We didn't see her when she came in, but, after that first evening, David's visits to the convent became more frequent, and Chummy went out more. She didn't say anything, to our keen disappointment, but became quieter and less of a good-old-chum, jolly-old-chum type of girl. We tried probing, of course, but the most we could get out of her was that 'Police work is very interesting. Much wider and more varied and interesting than you would think.'

'Anything else?' we asked, eagerly.

'What else?' she enquired innocently.

'Well . . . anything . . . sort of . . . interesting?'

'I've told him about my plans to be a missionary, if that's what you mean.'

We sighed deeply. It was hopeless. If all they ever talked about was the Metropolitan Police and missionaries, what future could there be? Poor old Chummy. Perhaps her mater was right, and she really was on the shelf.

It was another of those rush times. We were flying about. Eleven deliveries in two days and nights, postnatal visits, an antenatal clinic, lectures to attend, and the telephone constantly ringing.

I was on first call, and thankful to be resting after a hectic night and day with no sleep. The phone rang. Wearily I picked it up.

'My wife's in labour. She told me to call the midwife.'

Hastily I collected my bag and looked at the duty rota to see who would now be on first call. Chummy's name was at the top of the list. I ran to her room and banged on the door.

'Chummy! I'm going out. You're on first call.'

There was no response. I banged again and burst into the room.

'You're on first—'

My voice trailed away, and I backed off, abashed, guilty of an unforgivable intrusion; it was one of those things you should never, ever do. Chummy was in bed with her policeman.

Chapter Seventeen

THE WEDDING

Chummy married her policeman and she also became a missionary. Mrs Fortescue-Cholmeley-Browne, her mater, tried to organise a society wedding, with a reception at the Savoy Hotel, but Chummy refused. 'You owe it to your family, dear,' she said, applying the pressure. Still she refused. She wanted a simple wedding in our local church, All Saints, to be conducted by our local rector, with a reception in the church hall. 'But we cannot announce in *The Times* that the reception will be in a church hall in the East India Dock Road!' Mater exclaimed in alarm. 'And what about photographs? I will have to inform *Tatlers* and *Society News*. The family expect it. We can't have the reporters and photographers coming to a church hall, of all things.'

But Chummy was adamant: no announcements, no photographers.

Next came the issue of a wedding dress. Mater wanted to take her to Norman Hartnell, the Queen's dressmaker, for a wedding gown. Chummy refused, even more emphatically. She wasn't going to be dressed up like a Christmas tree fairy. 'But you must, dear. We are all dressed by Hartnell.' No, she wouldn't budge. She would wear a tailored suit. 'But you must wear white, dear. Virginal white for a wedding.'

'I'm not entitled to,' replied Chummy wickedly. That put a stop to any further entreaties.

The wedding party left from Nonnatus House, and I am not at all sure that the Reverend Mother would have approved of the disruption it caused had she seen it. But she was far away in Chichester, so it did not matter. The Sisters were in a real flutter of excitement because nothing like this had ever happened in the convent, and we girls were in a state bordering on panic trying to get ready. Mrs B had been baking all week and was putting the finishing touches to delectable dishes on the last morning, but Fred the boiler man had to go into her kitchen to attend to the boiler, which nearly drove her wild, and we all thought she would walk out. Sister Julienne sorted them out and calmed the cook, which was just as well, because without her the reception would have been a flop.

Amid all the flurry of preparation, the routine work had to be dealt with. We each had our usual list of ante- or postnatal visits, babies to bathe, feeding to be supervised, and so on. In addition, the general district nursing, especially the insulin injections, had to be attended to.

The day started badly for Trixie because she had washed and set her hair first thing and had then gone out on her bike to do her visits, so her hair was blown about, and when she got back it looked a mess. She kept wailing, 'What am I going to do with my hair? It's all over the place, and I can't do a thing with it!' Cynthia advised Vitapointe and gave her a tube, but Trixie in her hurry picked up a tube of foundation cream, which she smothered all over her hair. So then her hair was covered in grease, which looked a great deal worse. Cynthia advised washing it again.

'But it's too late. I can't go to a wedding with wet hair,' Trixie cried.

'Well, you certainly can't go to a wedding with pink face cream on your hair!'

Preparations started in earnest. A face pack was essential, then toning lotion; nails buffed and polished. Stockings were missing, or not matching, or laddered. A skirt had to be ironed.

'Be careful. It's too hot.'

'But I can't turn it down.'

'You'll have to leave it to get cooler.'

'I haven't time.'

'You'll have to. It will ruin the skirt if it's too hot.'

'Stupid thing. Why don't we get a better one?'

Hair clips had to be found, curlers taken out, lipsticks swapped, perfumes sniffed.

'I think I like the Musk.'

'The Freesia is more suitable for a wedding.'

'It's too light.'

'Well, the Musk is too heavy.'

'No, it's not. Don't be such a misery.'

Eyes are the window to the soul, they tell us. But that was not good enough for us girls. Eyes needed serious embellishment. Eyebrows had to be plucked, eyelashes curled, eyeshadow blended, eyeliner drawn with trembling haste, mascara . . .

'Damn!'

'What's up?'

'This mascara's dried out.'

'Spit on it, then.'

'That's disgusting.'

'No, it's not. Keeps it moist. Here have some of mine.'

'Not if you've been spitting on it, thank you very much.'

'Please yourself.'

Trixie had decided that the only thing to do was to wash her hair again, and now she was frantically trying to dry it.

'This stupid dryer is useless. Haven't we got a better one?'

'I'll get mine.'

'Yours blows too hard. I tried it before.'

'Beggars can't be choosers.'

Accessories required careful thought. A brooch was pinned on, then taken off, a necklace tried, earrings swapped, bracelets considered. Scarves had to be compared.

'That one matches your dress, you know.'

'I think I prefer this one. It's a contrast.'

'No. Bit too dominant. Try that one over there.'

'How does that look?'

'Better, much better. I like it.'

'OK, then I'll wear it. No, I won't. The silly thing will only get in the way. I won't wear a scarf at all.'

The only person who wasn't rushing wildly around preparing for the wedding was the bride herself. Chummy was perfectly calm and composed, and quietly smiling at the rest of us in our excitement.

'You sort yourselves out,' she said. 'I'm all ready. I will just go along the corridor and spend half an hour by myself in the chapel until it's time to go across the road to the church.'

One thing that had to be resolved was who should remain behind to be on call. Sister Julienne was adamant that we girls should all attend the wedding ceremony *and* the reception, so then came the discussion about which of the Sisters should remain at Nonnatus House.

'Weddings are for the young,' said Sister Evangelina. 'I'll stay behind.'

'No, no. That wouldn't be fair,' chorused her Sisters. 'We know you would like to go. We'll do a rota, and take it in turns.'

So that is what they did.

We left for the church, walked down the war-damaged road, past the bomb site that had been St Frideswide's Church, round the corner, across the East India Dock Road to All Saints Church on the south side of the road. No cars, no flowers, no bridesmaids – nothing like that. We could have been going out for an afternoon stroll. Chummy was wearing a simple grey suit, flat shoes, no make-up, no hat. She looked her usual self, but somehow more than herself, more than the Chummy we had grown to love.

The social division in the church was conspicuous. The Fortescue-Cholmeley-Brownes, oozing class, sat on one side of the aisle, and the Thompsons, shouting suburbia, sat on the other. We sat on Chummy's side with the nuns and several nurses from St Thomas's Hospital. On David's were half a dozen strapping young policemen. The policemen only came because David was popular, and for the chance of free beer. Also, they were intrigued. What on earth was a girl who wanted to be a missionary going to be like? And what, in the name of all that was holy, could they expect of a wedding party put on by a group of nuns?

They entered the church and were directed to David's side, where they sat self-consciously among the Thompson relatives. But when a crowd of young nurses entered in their wide skirts, their tight waists and high-heeled shoes, and sat down on Chummy's side, their spirits soared. They couldn't believe their luck and tried leaning sideways in the pews to make eye contact with nods and grins. But the girls ignored them, of course.

The nurses from St Thomas's had come because they found it hard to believe that Chummy was getting married at all. They had been convinced that she was firmly on the shelf, destined for a worthy spinsterhood. They were also, I'm sorry to say, condescending. 'Is it true that she's marrying a policeman, my dear? With all her connections, surely she could have done better than that? She must have been desperate, that's all I can say.' They sat demurely among the Fortescue-Cholmeley-Brownes, aware that a group of young men on the other side were trying to attract their attention, but deliberately turning their pretty heads to study the Stations of the Cross adjoining the opposite wall. The air was charged with testosterone, but the flirting had to be suppressed when Chummy entered on the arm of her father.

The wedding ceremony was beautiful, the love between these two like-minded young people filling the church with a golden light. Before God, and the present congregation, they pledged their lifelong vows to each other and stepped out into the sunshine as man and wife.

At the reception the policemen made straight for the young nurses, who rapidly forgot their hoity-toity airs and graces. Everything looked set fair for a good old party. The Fortescue-Cholmeley-Brownes lined up for the ceremonial hand-shaking and introductions, but the Thompsons didn't know what to do and stood around looking sheepish, until Chummy rescued them with, 'Oh come on, Mater, let's not bother with all that. Let's just mix. It will be much nicer.'

Mater's face, half hidden by an exquisite hat, looked a trifle sour. She approached Mrs Thompson, David's mother.

'Are you related to the Baily-Thompsons of Wiltshire?'

'No.'

'Ah! Well – er – perhaps to the Thompson-Bretts of India?'

'I don't think so.'

'Well, you might be, you know. It was a large family.'

'I couldn't rightly say, madam. I don't know that any of my relations has been abroad. We come from Battersea, and we were all in trade.'

'Oh, really? How very interesting.'

'Yes. We have a nice little place, with a nice garden. Just right for a little child to run around in. You must come and have tea with me some day.'

'Enchanted.' With a pained smile, the lady inclined her head.

'And when we have grandchildren, we'll see a lot more of each other, I'm sure.'

'Oh, no doubt, no doubt. Delightful talking to you, Mrs Thompson.'

And the poor lady crossed the social divide to talk with her own set about the shortcomings of the other side.

Colonel Fortescue-Cholmeley-Browne, in grey tails and

topper, opened conversation with Mr Thompson, in Moss Bros wedding hire and trilby.

'I say, old chap, let's have a snort together.'

'Don't mind if I do. You're paying for it.'

'Well, er, yes. Customary, you know. Noblesse oblige. Father of the bride, and all that.'

'And I'm father of the groom, so that makes us related, in a way.'

'Related!'

'Well, in a way.'

'I hadn't thought of it like that, I must say. Tell me a bit about yourself. I'm India, ex-army. Were you in the services?'

'Well, yes, sir. I was staff orderly to the officers of the Third Riflemen's Division, East Sussex, in the First World War.'

'Staff orderly?'

'Yes, sir.'

'How interesting. How frightfully interesting.'

The colonel did not look at all interested. Soon he crossed the room to join his wife.

'Not a pukka sahib in the whole room. No one worth talking to.'

'She's really let us down. We never could take her anywhere, and I'm quite sure we never will. I suppose I must go round and "mix" with her friends, as she puts it, but it will be the last time, I assure you. I think I will talk to that old lady sitting by herself over there.'

The old lady was Sister Monica Joan, who was fully absorbed with a dish of jelly and blancmange. Mrs Fortescue-Cholmeley-Browne approached her graciously.

'Can I introduce myself?'

Sister Monica Joan looked up sharply.

'Induce yourself? What! Induce yourself? My good woman, let it be known that I do not at all approve of inducing. A baby should come naturally, and the vast majority will, without the need for all these inductions. And what is a woman of your age doing being pregnant? It's indecent. And now you are asking me if you can induce yourself. Are you planning an abortion? Is that what? I tell you, it's illegal, and I'll have nothing to do with it. Be off with you.'

Poor Mater, shaken to the core, returned to her husband's side.

'I'm never going to get over this, never,' she murmured.

'Stiff upper lip, old girl,' retorted the colonel. 'This can't last for long, and then they're going to Sierra Leone, I understand.'

'Thank God for that. Best place for her,' said Mater emphatically.

Sister Julienne was quietly thrilled at the way Chummy had developed. Many girls had come to Nonnatus House aspiring to be medical missionaries, but somehow Chummy would always stand out in her mind. She gazed at the tall, happy girl standing at the other side of the room and fondly remembered her awkwardness when she first came to the convent, falling over things or walking into stationary objects. Above all she remembered Chummy learning to ride a bike with that nice boy Jack helping her. That was when the girl's true mettle first became apparent – she was indomitable. Sister Julienne chuckled to herself as she looked across the room at David, the policeman Chummy had somehow managed to run into and almost knock unconscious. So this was how the Good Lord had planned it!

Sister Julienne smiled around her at the happy faces, at Mrs B, in her element amid all the catering, Fred ambling around, moving chairs, clearing up, and obviously making wisecracks for the benefit of all. She looked across at the nurses from St Tommy's, who were roaring with laughter at the policemen, and thought how delightful it was to see young people enjoying themselves. And then her gaze fell on the frigid face of Mrs

Fortescue-Cholmeley-Browne. This isn't right, she thought. I must go over and have a word with her.

After the usual pleasantries, Sister Julienne went straight to the point.

'Mothers and daughters seldom understand each other.'

'What makes you say a thing like that?' said Mrs Fortescue-Cholmeley-Browne guardedly.

'Experience.'

'Experience? You have no children.'

'No, but I have a family. I am one of a family of nine, and I saw the tension between my mother and her five daughters. None of us lived up to her expectations. She did not attend any of their weddings. Not one! And when I took religious vows, she was outraged. I was embarrassing the family, she said. So you see, I know all about misunderstandings between mothers and daughters.'

Mrs Fortescue-Cholmeley-Browne sat silent. She was not going to be drawn. After a moment's pause, Sister went on.

'Camilla is a fine young woman. You can be very proud of her. She has the makings of nobility in her. She has strength of character, steadfast pursuit of her goal and, above all, mental and physical courage. These are the qualities that built the British Empire.'

Sister Julienne had scored a goal. Mrs Fortescue-Cholmeley-Browne came from a colonial family. Her father had been official adviser to the Raj and administrator of Bengal. Her husband, the Governor of Rajasthan. She knew all about the qualities that had built the British Empire. After a pause, she said, 'Well, I wish I could see it.'

'You will, I assure you. Mothers and daughters always draw closer to each other as the years pass. Camilla and David—'

Mrs Fortescue-Cholmeley-Browne butted in: 'This David! This fellow she is marrying. A common policeman. I ask you! What sort of marriage is that?'

'He may be a common policeman, but I have every reason to believe he is a fine young man and will make a good husband. He has a heroic war record. He flew and landed behind the German lines at Arnhem, you know, and not only survived, but helped others to survive.'

'I didn't know that.' The lady's face softened.

'No. Probably not. It is not the sort of thing he talks about.'

The time for speeches was drawing near. Sister Julienne felt she had no more than a few minutes alone with the mother of the bride, and must introduce some humour into the situation.

'Another thing. For years after he was demobbed from the army, David's father—' she pointed to Mr Thompson '—strongly disapproved of his son. Nothing the boy could do was good enough for Mr T. So you see, the same misunderstandings and tensions can arise between fathers and sons. Often worse. The son does not live up to the father's expectations and earns his reproaches. And when he does succeed, very often masculine rivalry can set in as the father desperately tries to beat his son at the very game he has initiated.'

For the first time that day, Mrs Fortescue-Cholmeley-Browne burst out laughing. Chummy, who had been watching her mother apprehensively, looked across the room with amazement.

'Oh, how true. I know that syndrome all too well. My own husband shows a deadly rivalry with our son over sculling. The boy's far better than him, but he can't or won't see it. He is taking extra training courses and comes back exhausted, hardly able to move a muscle, and needs physiotherapy. He'll injure his back, or something, before he will admit defeat. I can't tell you what the atmosphere is like in our house sometimes with these two men competing against each other.'

The two ladies looked at each other, nearly creasing themselves with laughter but suppressing their giggles because the speeches were just about to start. Sister managed to whisper, 'I know *exactly* what you mean.'

The wedding speeches were predictable and charming. The colonel spoke with affection of his only daughter and said he was proud of her nursing career. We girls clapped and shouted, 'Hear, hear!' The best man said that David was a credit to the force, and Sierra Leone would be lucky to get him, and the policemen stamped and cheered.

The boys from the South Poplar Youth Club band arrived, and with them came a wedding guest who had been invited to the church but had not come. We had all wondered why. This was Jack, a local lad of about thirteen who had been instrumental in teaching Chummy to ride a bicycle when she first came to Nonnatus House. A close bond had developed between Chummy and Jack, and she had been surprised and a little sad that he had not come to her wedding. When he walked in, slightly behind the other boys, she shouted out, 'Jack! You've come – I'm so glad,' and rushed over to him. In her exuberance she would probably have taken him in her arms, but he quickly backed off with a 'Steady on, miss, steady on.' So she shook hands in the manner that boys of that age prefer. It would not do to shame him in front of the other lads.

Mrs B had held back a substantial part of the feast for the boys from the SPY Club, knowing that it would be necessary, and while they were all tucking in, Chummy managed a few words with Jack.

'Well, I wouldn't miss your weddin', miss, but I didn't wanna come wiv all them toffs, like, so I comes wiv the lads, like, an' I gotta presen' for yer, miss. I made it in metalwork at school.'

He pulled a brown paper package from his pocket and thrust it furtively into her hands, making sure that his back was turned to the others so that they couldn't see. 'It's fer you, miss.'

Then he turned quickly and blended in with the other lads.

Chummy returned to her husband and opened the parcel. It was a tiny bicycle, carefully constructed out of wire and metal.

The SPY club band started up, somewhat out of tune but with plenty of rhythm, and the happy couple led the dancing. At seven o'clock, they left to get the night train to Cornwall, where they were spending their honeymoon. A taxi came to take them to Paddington station, and a big crowd gathered outside the church hall to wish them well and see them off. Jack didn't stand waving with the rest of us. He ran round to the back of the hall, grabbed his bicycle and gave chase to the taxi, with Chummy and David looking out of the rear window in astonishment. He was a strong boy and fast. He followed the taxi all the way and was on the platform to wave them off as the train steamed out of Paddington station.

Chummy married her policeman and she also became a missionary. Together they went to Sierra Leone, where she opened the first midwifery service at the mission station and ran the small hospital. David joined the police and became a senior officer in the force. They found the work harder and more demanding than they could ever have imagined, but they had the strength of youth and idealism to carry them through. Above all, they had the love to support and sustain each other in times of crisis. They stayed in Africa throughout their lives, and Chummy and I corresponded for a few years. They had a family, but she continued her work in a teaching capacity. She must have been desperately busy, and in the circumstances it is not easy to continue writing letters indefinitely to an old nursing colleague. We exchanged Christmas cards for a few years, but eventually they petered out. She was a unique character, and it was a happiness and a privilege to have known her.

PART VIII

FRED

In which Fred rents a plot

And now we come to the main body of the new material: the allotment story. All of Fred's previous little earners have failed for one reason or another, with the exception of pig breeding, in which, with Sister Julienne's invaluable help, he is surprisingly successful. For the first time we discover Fred had a surname! As far as I was concerned, Fred was just Fred, but no, his surname was Wagstaff. Who would have thought? The allotment story completes Fred's story and is a fitting conclusion to the book.

Chapter Eighteen

THE MUDCHUTE ALLOTMENTS

Those who have not experienced at first hand the passions that burn in the hearts of allotment holders have missed a rare treat in life. Let a man rent from his local council a pole, or even just half a pole of ground, for the purpose of growing his vegetables, and he becomes overnight a duke, nay a prince, the owner of endless rolling acres of verdant pastures. Gone from his mind are unworthy preoccupations with the dogs or the Derby, with pubs or parties. More lofty thoughts prevail these days; thoughts of succulent lettuce in springtime, ripe tomatoes in autumn, healthy spinach for the children's bones. There is nothing he cannot grow in the winter days, sitting beside his fire thumbing through seed catalogues, comparing prices, making lists and endless notes about rotation of crops and soil conditions and fertilisers.

With the advent of spring weather he is out early and late, with his wellies and spade, digging over his pole or half-pole preparatory to the planting season. Scores of other allotment holders are also out in this fine spring weather, digging their plots. And this is where the fun and the trouble start.

Each allotment is very close to its neighbour, and a spirit of neighbourliness might or might not prevail between the registered holders of adjacent plots divided only by a narrow path no more than the width of a wheelbarrow. Two men holding neighbouring plots might enjoy each other's company. But two men who dislike each other, and in each of whose bosoms the passion for vegetable growing burns fiercely, can nurture a quiet resentment of the very existence and proximity of the other, which can be fanned into murderous hatred if the circumstances dictate.

Let no one suppose that a community of interests makes for peace and tranquillity in human affairs. If this were so, the flower ladies' circle or the amateur dramatics group would be havens of sweetness and light, and we all know that they are not.

The digging goes silently on. The men who tolerate each other's company amicably might exchange a companionable grunt now and then, or a brief word about the tilth or the slugs – the interest in slugs is inexhaustible. But the men who dislike each other dig in grim silence, back to back, but each keeping a careful sideways eye on the other, anxious that he should not be outshone in any way. It is hard to imagine how anyone could be outshone in a simple matter like digging, but be assured that subtle standards of perfection prevail, to which each aspires, to the deepest chagrin of the other.

Planting commences in April and May. Furrows are furrowed, seeds are scattered, and markers mark each careful row. Weeds are weeded, tender cabbages are tenderly watered, and wayward bean shoots are taught how to climb their bean poles. Activity is intense, and passions run high when the lettuces are devoured by slugs, the cabbages by caterpillars, and the carrots by carrot flies.

This is when the two men who dislike each other begin silently and secretly to blame each other for their individual losses and failures. Neither can bear to think the loss or failure could be of his own making, or simply the vagaries of nature. No, indeed, that other fellow has been picking caterpillars off his cabbages and putting them on to mine! Villainy! He must be taught a lesson. I'll teach him. I'll pick them off and put them back!

Surprising as it may seem, grown men, from bank managers to bar tenders, from consultant surgeons to cab drivers, behave in this manner on millions of allotments all over the country. And it was no different on the Mudchute allotments on the Isle of Dogs.

The Mudchute allotments used to be beautiful, a haven of green and birdsong in the midst of the noise, the boats, cranes and warehouses of the greatest port in the world. The allotments covered an area of roughly ten acres divided into about one hundred plots of a pole or half a pole each. They were right on the water's edge, and those fortunate to possess a plot adjoining the Thames could hear the sound of the lapping water all the time as they worked. The allotments were the last little piece of rural land remaining from the time when the Isle of Dogs was a marsh used mainly for cattle grazing, whereon dwelled in scattered hamlets a small population of people who called themselves the Islanders. In the nineteenth century, industrialisation began. The great Millwall, East India and West India Docks were dug, tens of thousands of men poured in for the employment afforded by the maritime trading, and the tenements were built to house the dockers and their families. Life for the Islanders changed irrevocably, but the allotments remained their possession, courtesy of the council, and they were continuously in use.

The soil was rich and fertile, and, due to the proximity of the Thames, never dried out in summer. Many families lived on an abundant supply of fresh vegetables, which did much to improve the health of the children. Some of the men had erected chicken coops and kept fowls, which provided eggs and meat. Keeping chickens on the allotments was an easy matter, because they ate a lot of the waste vegetation and were not plagued by the foxes, the public enemy of chickens. Not surprisingly, there were no foxes on the Isle of Dogs. The allotment holders had only one problem – manure, or rather the want of it.

Manure is the first essential of vegetable growing. Without it, beans will fail to climb, potatoes will be small and stunted, and vegetable marrows will not stand a chance. Chicken manure is good but there is not really enough of it to spread thickly, and the same can be said of compost, which the men produced from their own waste vegetation. In the 1930s there was a dairy in Stepney, so an abundant supply of cow manure was available, but the dairy closed down in that decade. In the 1950s a good many dray horses still worked, especially for coal merchants and the breweries, but the horses were not stabled on the Isle of Dogs. Men could not take their wheelbarrows and just fill them up with well-rotted horse manure, which as we all know is the very best manure obtainable at any price. No, they had to order it from stables far away in Essex, which was inconvenient and, as the years went by, increasingly expensive. Something had to be done about the manure problem.

Chapter Nineteen

FRED RENTS A PLOT

Fred had been boiler man and odd-job man at Nonnatus House for many years, and some of his activities were very odd indeed, assuming, of course, that his outrageous stories were to be believed. Whoever heard of a 'cooper's barrel bottom knocker', or of a freelance fireworks maker? I never knew whether he was having us on or not as we sat around the large wooden table in the kitchen, having our breakfast, while Fred stoked his boiler and told us his tall stories. After many years of reflecting on Fred's extraordinary characteristics, I am inclined to think he was not pulling a fast one. I certainly witnessed the collapse of his quails enterprise and his toffee apple empire when the two got mixed up and quail feathers became stuck to his toffee apples and the public health authorities forbade the continuance of both activities.

After that Fred, with the invaluable help of Sister Julienne, turned to pig breeding. He kept a sow in the backyard of his little cottage in Cubitt Town and the litters she produced afforded a steady income for the odd-job entrepreneur. Everything went well for about a year. Blossom was serviced by a magnificent stud boar and the piglets kept on coming. The neighbours did not seem to object to a pig in the backyard adjoining theirs, and the smells were no worse than the river smells to which they were long habituated. When the mess got to be too much, Fred just shovelled some of it up and tipped it in the river. All the best pig breeders would say that you cannot possibly keep a pig in such conditions, but Fred proved them wrong. He was highly successful.

One fine evening, Fred was enjoying a cooling pint in his local when a fragment of conversation caught his attention.

'Can't ge' it, not fer no money yer can't.'

'My dad go' cows muck, afore the War. Kept 'im goin nicely, 'e says.'

'Cows, you can keep yer cows. It's good 'orse shit as wha' I'm after.'

'I'm tellin' yer, I'd take any ol' shit.'

Fred moved closer.

'Yeah, I'm wiv yer. Bu' where to ge' it. That's wha' I wants to know.'

'Truman is movin' 'is 'orses, an' all.'

'No!'

'Straigh' up. Goin' to Essex, they says.'

'When?'

'Search me. I'm regular pissed off, I can tell you. Good 'orse shit is wha' I likes best – an' now 'e's goin' to Essex!'

Fred had a particular knack of opening conversation with strangers. He was a singular looking man, no more than five feet two inches tall, thin as a bit of string, all sinews and bones, which seemed to stick out at odd angles, one solitary yellow tooth in the middle of his front upper jaw, a roll-up fag perpetually stuck to his lower lip and the most spectacular squint you have ever seen. He sidled up to the men in his sideways fashion and looked up with his north-east eye at the man who was standing; the men who were seated he was able to look down upon with his south-east eye, so that each man, standing or sitting, had the impression he was being looked at.

'If I may insinuate myself into your company, gents, wivout aspersions, am I righ' in finking you was lookin' for a nice drop o' shit?'

'Yep, yer right.'

'Well, let's all 'ave anuvver drink, 'cos I reckons as 'ow I can 'elp you.'

'In tha' case, barman, bring us all a drink, will you?' What're you having?'

'Thank you kindly, very civil of you. Mine's a beer. Nah then, wha' was it we was talkin' about?'

Fred looked around him blandly, and started whistling through his tooth. They reminded him. Fred made a great show of jerking his memory back to the subject under discussion.

'Ah yes, shit. That was it. Would you gents be interested in a nice drop o' pig shit?'

'Can you ge' it?'

'Where?'

'How much?'

'Pig shit? You can keep yer pig shit. It's 'orse shit is wha' I'm after.'

'Well, you go to Essex for it, mate. Where's this 'ere pig shit?'

'Cubitt Town.'

'How much?'

'Two bob a wheel barrer load.'

'Done.'

They shook hands all round and turned their attention to sipping their beer.

And that is how Fred came to supply the Mudchute allotments with much-needed manure.

Two of the men came to Fred's house with their barrows the next evening and loaded up. They arrived the next day, with a couple more chaps, and then more turned up with their barrows. Within a fortnight Fred's pile was exhausted.

We girls and Fred discussed the matter over breakfast. Fred was speaking.

'Trouble is, one pig and 'er litter ain't enough for the allotments. It needs about six pigs fer that.'

'Well, can't you get some more porkers, old chap?' Chummy said.

'But where'm I gonna keep 'em?'

'No room in the backyard, then?'

'Nope.'

Cynthia spoke for the first time.

'Well, why not keep them on the allotments? There's plenty of room there.'

Fred jumped up from his position on the floor beside the boiler, ran over to Cynthia and kissed her, an experience not easily forgotten.

'Brilliant, yer brillian', my girl. I'll rent an allotment, and keep pigs. Other people keep chickens and rabbits on their plots, so I'll keep pigs on mine.'

That same afternoon, Fred went round to the Poplar Council offices, an imposing building in Poplar High Street, to enquire about taking an allotment. The council lady was very helpful. She brought out a hand-drawn plan, which looked like nothing intelligible, covered in squares, all of which were numbered, and a few of which were coloured red. She explained that it was a plan of the allotments, and that the red squares marked the free plots, available for rental. She suggested that Fred should go to the site and choose one of them.

It was all very bewildering, because when he got there none of the plots were numbered, as the plan clearly suggested they should be, and none of the shapes of the plots seemed to correspond with the shapes drawn on the plan. But Fred was not a fool, and as he wandered around, enjoying the sunshine and the sounds of the river, he figured out that a plot, carefully hoed and planted, was the possession of a proud owner, whereas a plot covered in weeds would be free. Eventually he chose one in a corner with a fence on two sides, which would be helpful for him when he constructed his pigsty. He returned to the council offices, paid a nominal sum of five shillings for a year, and became the proud owner of a plot on the Mudchute allotments.

Chapter Twenty

THE PIGSTIES ARE CONSTRUCTED

It would be an understatement to say that Sister Julienne was interested in Fred's latest enterprise. Since her profession into the religious life, there had not been a lot of opportunity for contact with the porcine race, and she was quietly thrilled by Fred's activities. She had, of course, been instrumental in the beginning, and I doubt if Fred's enterprise would have succeeded at all without her knowledge and practical help.

Many were her duties: Sister in Charge of Nonnatus House, responsible for the spiritual welfare of her Sisters and Novices, and for the smooth continuance of the daily offices and the liturgical life of the convent – all this would have been enough for any ordinary woman. But, in addition, she practised a full professional life as nurse and midwife, taught her students, went out each day on her bicycle to her patients in the district, and accepted her place on the rota of night calls. Yet, nonetheless, she managed to find the time to visit Blossom in Fred's backyard, to assess her happiness and welfare, and to have a little chat with her.

It was apparent that the pig knew and responded to Sister Julienne, because she grunted and humphed and ambled out of her sty whenever Sister approached with a bunch of carrots or some turnip tops in hand. The sow rubbed herself against the wood, allowing her back to be scratched, and lifted her snout with sensuous pleasure to Sister's caressing hand. Whenever a litter of piglets was born, Sister would be among the first to be there, admiring and talking to the proud mother in words that only a pig can understand.

On the corner plot of the allotments, with the energy that characterised Fred when he was on to something, four pigsties were constructed. Cost was next to nothing, because the importation of timber was a considerable part of the trading in the docks, and huge timber yards existed. Fred had no difficulty in getting as many offcuts as he wanted.

One of the men he had met in the pub was Chip, a carpenter by trade, who worked in one of the yards. Having benefited from the manure, Chip had a vested interest in the development of the pigsties, and brought the offcuts to the allotments on his barrow each evening. His knowledge of how to handle wood and how to construct virtually anything out of wood ensured that the sties were well built, which they would not have been if slapdash Fred had done the job alone. Chip was a quiet, thoughtful sort of man, and it was a perfect relationship – Fred did all the talking and Chip did all the work.

The other men on the allotments watched the progress with interest. Many of them thought that hen houses were under construction, and Chip encouraged this idea, advising Fred that until the pigs were installed it would be better to say nothing of their intention. Fred, who was inclined to be a big mouth and a boaster, was all for letting everyone, including the council, know his plans, but Chip advised against it. He pointed out that it was not certain that the council would allow pigs on the allotments. He'd had a look at the Rules for Allotment Holders and could see only rules about 'wooden constructions', which must not be more than six feet high. Well, he wasn't going up more than six feet, was he, and the Rules didn't say nuffink about what was kept in 'em. If the council didn't know nuffink, they couldn't say nuffink. This seemed to be sound advice. Fred was thinking of the expansion of his empire, and all the money that would be coming in. Chip was thinking of his prize beans, which he intended showing at the Dulwich Horticultural Show, and for which the manure would be a necessary prerequisite. Both men worked steadily on.

Three weeks later, Blossom was installed in her new home, which, by any standards, was a great improvement on the old one. She had a well-constructed sty, more room to move around and plenty of opportunity for rooting. Any surveyor who knew his job would describe it as a desirable residence in a favoured area. The other men on the allotments were intrigued. Many of them came over to the sty to stare down at Blossom happily munching cabbage stalks, whilst others maintained an aloof distance. All were interested in their own ways. One was heard to mutter, 'Well, I ain't so sure as 'ow keeping pigs is allowed,' but he was silenced by the majority who reckoned you could do what you liked on your plot and who's to say you couldn't?

It so happened that Blossom was heavily pregnant, and a litter of piglets was born a week or so later. Interest was renewed, and word got round, and the wives of the allotment holders brought their children to see the family of fourteen, contentedly suckling their massive milky mother. The children talked about it at school, and the local schoolmistress brought her class of thirty children to see them. None of the children had seen a pig, except in picture books, and it was considered to be of great educational benefit to them. Word got round even faster now, and by the weekend two more classes of thirty children had paid a visit to Blossom.

The men on the allotments were accustomed to a quiet life. One of the joys of allotment holding, as indeed it is with fishing, is that you can get away from the wife and kids. To have all these children runnin' around, screamin' an' 'ollerin' created a certain amount of discontent, but this was brushed aside when it became clear that the manure supplies would be multiplied fourteenfold. Piglets grow fast and the men were soon coming to Fred with their barrows for two bob's worth, and the beans and brussels and leeks were responding with verdant profusion.

Fred decided to keep three of the sows for breeding, and to sell the rest for bacon. Sister Julienne had been asked to pick out the best breeding sows, because Fred wasn't sure himself; they all looked much the same to him. Sister's visits to the allotments when the piglets were newborn had been an occasion of surprise, and given rise to comment amongst the men; but when the little nun and Fred were seen side by side in deep and earnest conversation, hanging over the edge of the sty, poking the piglets with sticks and singling three of them out for closer examination, their surprise and interest were renewed. When Sister put on a pair of wellington boots, hitched up her habit and girdle and climbed over the side to examine the piglets' eyes, ears, teeth and backsides, they leaned on their spades and left off work. The three sows that were selected Fred named Blackberry, Bluebell and Chrystaline.

As the summer days matured, the three young sows matured too, and the stud boar from Essex was hired to do his stuff. More piglets arrived, and with that came more manure – the vegetables increased in size to prize-winning proportions. Chip the carpenter had always been keen on beans, and had regularly produced runners twelve inches long, which had frequently been decorated with a second- or third-prize rosette at the Dulwich Horticultural Show.

His neighbouring plot was owned by Nobby, a 'miserable old sod' (if we are to trust Chip's judgement) who never had a civil word for anyone and who had 'a right nasty streak in him'. He, too, was keen on beans. For years both men had taken second and third prizes at the Dulwich show, and both men craved first prize. Having started to add manure to his soil early, Chip's beans were coming on a treat. Nobby, the neighbour, had held aloof from the pig manure, partly because he didn't want Chip to think that he, Nobby, was copying him, and partly because he didn't hold with pigs on the allotments, anyway. Nobby was using a patent fertiliser that came in powder form, which claimed to produce beans as long as yer arm and in which he had great faith.

Alas for Nobby, as the weeks passed it became clear that the manure had the edge. Vainly did he spread the powder, spray the leaves, weed around the roots, but all to no avail. Day by day anyone could see that Chip's beans were fuller, firmer and longer. Greatly was Nobby tempted to sneak up to Chip's trellis and pull off the best of the beans, but he knew that if he did such a thing 'someone' would see, and 'someone' would not only report the outrage to Chip, but word would spread and his name would become muddier than the mud of the Mudchute allotments! Collective moral outrage might even force him to give up his plot altogether. Poor Nobby; envy and resentment are nasty things to go to bed with each night.

Chapter Twenty-One

THE LADY FROM THE COUNCIL

One fine summer's day, the lady from the council visited the allotments. She did not do this very often, being more involved with paperwork and the drawing of plans than visiting them. But it was a lovely day and she hadn't a lot to do that afternoon, so she thought she would take a look. It was all very pleasant and peaceful as she ambled around, admiring the neat edges, tut-tutting at the untidy ones, pausing to examine more closely this or that, stooping to peer into the chicken houses and listen to the contented cluck-clucking of the hens. There was no one around, because all the men were at work, and the noise from the docks seemed far away. The gentle sounds of a river steamer and the chirping of sparrows were all that could be heard. A couple of pigeons courting caused her to smile dreamily as she ambled along.

An unexpected sound caught her ears, and the lady from the council paused to listen. There was a sort of grunt, followed by squeaks and squeals. Greatly perplexed, the lady from the council hurried to the corner from where the sounds were coming. She was a little out of breath when she reached the corner plot, but her breath failed her completely when she looked over the wooden fence and saw a large sow snuffling around, and a very large number of piglets. She couldn't believe her eyes. In order to regain her breath, she leaned on the wooden structure and stared and stared at the apparition. And the longer she stared, the more enchanted she became by the family.

The sow was healthy and well fed. The sty was clean and swept. The water trough was full and the bran trough was half full. The sow was drinking silently from the water, her curly tail quivering with delight. Having taken her fill, she turned her head and looked straight into the eyes of the lady from the council and, with a companionable sort of grunt, ambled slowly over towards her. The piglets squealed and scattered in all directions, avoiding their mother's dainty feet.

Sows with a litter to protect can be very tricky, but this one was more inclined to assess the situation than to launch into an attack without provocation, and the two females stood sizing each other up for quite a few minutes. Eventually the sow came up to the fence, raised her snout, closed her eyes and grunted. The lady from the council tentatively put out her hand, and scratched the bristly hide. The sow grunted and her tail revolved at high speed. The lady from the council murmured, 'Oh you dear thing.' Then the sow gave another grunt, ambled over to the corner and lay down. The piglets rushed squealing and tumbling over each other to the milk bar so generously offered, and within seconds each one was sucking voraciously, eyes closed and tails whirling.

The lady from the council gazed with rapture at the blissful scene for several minutes. Eventually she reluctantly left the pastoral idyll that she had stumbled upon, and took the bus back to the council offices. It had been a pleasant afternoon, away from the dreary routine of her office job, and her mind was full of happy, dreamy thoughts as the bus rumbled along. She dozed off but was rudely awakened as, with a screech of brakes, the bus stopped with a jerk. The lady from the council woke up, confused and bewildered. What had happened? She looked out of the window, and the bus driver and a costermonger with his barrow stuck at an awkward angle across the road were shouting at each other. Nothing much then, she thought to herself, and settled back in her seat for another little doze.

But the jerk had banished sleep, and banished also her dream. A chilling thought had entered her mind, as chill as the north wind. Were pigs allowed on the allotments?

The lady from the council passed a sleepless night. Her conscience, as a loyal employee of the borough, told her that she must report the finding of pigs on the Mudchute allotments to her superiors; but her feminine intuition told her that if she did, they would put a stop to it.

Through the long and lonely hours of the silent night, she wrestled with the problem. What harm were pigs doing on the allotment? They were clearly of great benefit; they were well cared for, no one had complained and who was to say they should not be there anywhere? But a little worm niggled persistently at the back of her mind that someone would have something negative to say on the subject, and that someone might well be a senior council official upon whom she was dependent for her job. If he, Mr Mountshaft, got to know about the pigs, and learned that she had known about them and said nothing of the irregularity, not only would the pigs have to leave the allotments but she might have to leave the council. Her mother, who was getting on in years, frail and in poor health, depended on her. The clock struck three and the lady from the council could stay in bed no longer. She threw off the bedclothes – it was infernally hot, too hot to sleep – and thumped the pillow in anger. She put on her blue candlewick dressing gown and quietly (so as not to disturb her mother) crept downstairs and into their strip of garden, so lovingly tended by the two women.

A garden by night is completely different from a garden by day. The moon had gone and darkness surrounded her. She felt the great sleeping pulse of the city all around. Colour had gone from the fuchsias and the geraniums, but a perfume that she had not smelled before was rising from the damp earth. A small creature, probably a shrew, scampered near the fence, and a solitary bird gave a single call, and was silent. She sat down on the seat by the back door and leaned her aching head on the cool brickwork. What was she to do? What on earth was she to do?

It was high summer, when daybreak is early. A tinge of light from the east was changing the midnight-black sky to deepest purple, fast fading to violet-blue. The lady from the council dozed off on the garden chair and woke with a crick in the neck to find bright morning all around her. The solution had come in her sleep: she would thoroughly examine all the regulations and bye-laws relating to allotments and urban public lands. If keeping pigs on allotments was not prohibited, she would assume that it was permitted. If there were such a restriction, in writing, then reluctantly she would have to report her finding to Mr Mountshaft. Happy with this decision, she went upstairs to dress and prepare for work.

Chapter Twenty-Two

THE PIGS FLOURISH

Meanwhile, Fred's business ventures were thriving as never before. He had four breeding sows, with young pigs regularly going to market, and he had the sale, for hard cash, of manure to his fellow allotment holders. He worked early and late, feeding, watering and mucking out, and was bringing in more money than he had ever earned in a long life dedicated to 'little earners'. He could easily have afforded to quit his job as boiler man for the convent, but he did not do so. His affection for the Sisters was too great, he loved impressing us young girls with his tall stories, and, above all, his devotion to and reliance upon Sister Julienne was central to his life. It could perhaps be said that the little nun was the brains behind Fred's porcine enterprise, because he consulted her frequently about feed and suppliers and changes of mash as a sow came to parturition, or straw for bedding or space for piglets. Every word she uttered on the subject he carried out as though he were entrusted with the Holy Grail. The pigs flourished.

The summer was beautiful. Long, hot sunny days followed each other as though they would never end. It was the sort of summer when the English become almost Mediterranean in temperament. The allotment holders were in virtual heaven. With continuous sunshine, their cabbages were firming up, their peas were podding, their beans were fairly racing up the poles, the tiny, tender marrow plants were expanding with vast luxuriant leaves and displaying exquisite yellow flowers more lovely than a rose, more fragile than a lily, destined to die in a day, leaving tender little marrows on slender stems. The men were happy, and none happier than Chip, who could see himself as 'First Prize Winner for Beans' at the Dulwich Horticultural Show, perhaps with a gold medal for outstanding excellence.

But not all were happy. A minority of men had rejected the bounty showered from heaven, as it were, by the pigs, and each could see that his allotment was flourishing with less abundance than was the norm that year. Chief amongst the malcontents was Nobby, the morose plot holder next to Chip. Nobby could see (you'd have to be blind not to) that Chip's blasted beans were ten times better than his. He threw his patent bean fertiliser in the Thames and tore down his bean trellis. He'd forget the Dulwich show, wouldn't go near the damned thing. He fed what was left of his bean plants to his rabbits and sat by the river to contemplate, and to plan his revenge.

What he really wanted to do was to tear down Chip's beans, but it was out of the question – someone would see him doing it – eyes were everywhere, even in the middle of the night. No, he couldn't do that. He would have to attack his grievance at source. Nobby hurled a stone into the river and the splash gave him his idea. 'Attack at source.' That was it. Them damned pigs were the source of all his anger and frustration. If Chip hadn't got hold of all that pig shit, he, Nobby, would have been in with a chance at the Dulwich show. It was unfair competition, that's what it was. The pigs were the source of the trouble, and he would attack them. The more he thought about it, the more he convinced himself that pigs were not allowed on allotments. There had never been any before, so it stood to reason that they weren't allowed. He would consult with his fellow allotment holders, that's what he would do.

Resolutely he stomped up the central pathway to Plot 59,

held for approximately fifty-nine years by a chap devoted to marrows. To say that he had given his life, barring service in two world wars, to the cultivation of marrows would be no exaggeration. Plot 59 was a man set in his ways. For thirty-five years he had used cow dung from the Stepney milk herds, and when the cows were moved to Essex he had reluctantly transferred his custom to the stables belonging to the brewers. With the threat of the closure of the stables he had tried the patent packeted fertilisers, which promised miracles of verdant growth. At about the same time Fred had brought his pigs to the allotment, and most of the men were very excited about it, but, no, Plot 59 wouldn't give you a 'thank you' for pig shit. He'd paid good money for his patent fertiliser, and he was going to use it. He'd won first prize for marrows at the Dulwich Horticultural Show for as many years as he could remember, and he wasn't going to mess up his chances this year with pig shit 'what was too heavy and couldn't be broken up. Science is moving on all the time, and look what it says on the back of this 'ere packet about phosphorus and nitrogen! Makes you think, it do.'

Nobby approached Plot 59, who was contemplating the disaster of his marrows with sour and baleful malevolence. On Plot 58 there were marrow plants with leaves the size of dustbin lids and young marrows already forming. His marrows had hardly grown since they were planted out in early June, and pathetic little flowers had fallen off, sterile. Nobby sidled up to him.

'I don't 'old wiv no pigs on allotments, do you?'

'What?'

'Don't know wha' it's comin' to. Nex' fing, there'll be sheep and cows an' God knows wha' else.'

'Hmm . . .' No. 59 was a man of few words.

'We've never 'ad pigs on these allotments 'afore, 'ave we?'

'Nope.'

'Well, it can't be allowed then else we would 'ave 'ad 'em 'afore now.'

Nobby deemed it wise to say no more, but to leave Plot 59 with the wreck of his marrows, and the germ of an idea in his mind.

Over the next few weeks he went around several other malcontents who had so obviously failed to take advantage of Fred's provender, and whose vegetables were, as a result, suffering. With a word here and a word there, with a sideways look and a shrug, with a sneer of the lips and a hiss, he was able to build up a caucus of men who agreed that pigs were not allowed on the allotments, and it 'oughta be stopped, it did'.

Chapter Twenty-Three

ANCIENT RIGHTS

Although she had managed only a couple of hours sleep in an excruciating position, the lady from the council was clear in her head, and firm in her resolve as to what she had to do. She went to the council office early that morning. She selected from the files the bye-laws and regulations relating to allotments, which she carefully studied. She could find no reference to pigs, neither approving nor prohibiting the keeping of them on allotments. The only thing she found were regulations about wooden structures for keeping chickens or other small fowl, the size and proper construction of which was specified, but nothing more. Well, she mused, pigs were not chickens, but the structure of the pigsties was of high quality, and the size . . . ? Well, she would have to check the size to determine whether or not it fell within the regulations.

She went into the dusty basement to search for archive materials that might pertain to the subject. She found fascinating old maps and sketches and notes relating to the keeping of cows on the marshy swamps of the Isle of Dogs, and the rights of the Islanders to the free and unrestricted use of the pastureland. These marshy swamps had now become the docks, but the archives did not say what had become of the rights of the Islanders.

The lady from the council closed the file and took it upstairs. She hid it in the bottom drawer of her desk and put the key in her pocket. She was not a lawyer, merely a humble typist with a marked inferiority complex and a mother to support, but she was astute enough to see that if the Islanders had once owned the rights to keep livestock on the Isle of Dogs, and the rights had never been repealed, it could be argued that they, the Islanders, still retained those rights. The lady from the council was fundamentally a humble soul. She would never push herself forward, never argue and never presume above her station, as she put it. Many of her superiors in the council offices would have said that she was a doormat. But they would have been wrong. Like many people of her type, outwardly quiet and docile, she had a core of steel. Fair play was axiomatic to her creed. The Islanders had once owned the rights of the pastureland, and they had been stripped of them, apparently without a by-your-leave, or any legal process, in order to build the docks. The only open space that could resemble pasture-land was the allotments. If the Islanders owned the rights to pastureland, now called allotments, they would therefore have the right to keep cows or oxen or horses or any large animal, including pigs, on the allotments.

She would keep her own counsel and bide her time. If Mr Mountshaft found out about the pigs and tried to get them removed, she would produce the regulations and the archive material about ancient rights, and fight.

Having examined the regulations and bye-laws relating to allotments, the lady from the council had one further task to fulfil before she could satisfy herself that pigs were not precluded from allotments. She had to measure the size and structure of the pigsties. If they were too large or too high, or did not meet the council's requirements in any way, her conscience told her that she must inform Mr Mountshaft.

She could not go to the allotments during office hours, because Mr Mountshaft might ask where she was going and what she was doing. So she went after work. It was a lovely evening and again she was struck by the peace and tranquillity of the scene. She went straight to the corner where the pigs were housed. A small man was working amongst them. He was whistling a tuneless whistle, and, as he talked to his pigs, a damp fag swayed up and down on his lower lip.

'There's me beau'y. Done it again fer Daddy, eh?'

He scratched a large sow's snout and pulled her ears.

'They're lovely, they are, lovely as their mum, and you're the tops, my sweet'art.'

The pig appeared to appreciate his compliments, snorted and rubbed her head into his knees, nearly knocking him over. A litter of newborn piglets squealed and tumbled over each other, and the sow lay heavily down to feed them. The piglets were in frantic competition to get at the teats and pushed and fought ruthlessly, but soon each one was sucking vigorously, and peace was restored. Fred kneeled down to scratch the sow's nose and mutter words of endearment. She responded with contented grunts.

Fred took out his baccy and papers to roll another cigarette when he noticed a lady approaching. She did not realise that he had seen her because his back was towards her, but Fred's eyes were so singularly aligned that he could not see frontwards. He watched her with his north-east eye whilst rolling his fag.

'Oh, you sweet little things,' murmured the lady from the council, 'you pretty little things!'

'You likes pigs, then madam? I can tell you do. We got a lot in common, ma'am.'

Fred turned round and grinned, one yellow fang jutting over his lower lip, his eyes looking everywhere but at her. 'Are you one of them school teachers, ma'am? Don' mind me askin'?'

'No. I'm Miss Wilson from the council. I've come to measure your pigsties to be sure they meet the council's instructions about wooden buildings.'

Fred jerked upright. Mention of the council gave him an uneasy feeling. He had brushed aside the idea that pigs might not be allowed on allotments, but here was the council in person. Come spyin'!

'You wants 'a see Chip, ma'am. He made the sties, an' he knows all abaht it. Jes' you wait 'ere. I'll be right back.'

Fred climbed over the wall and ran down the pathways to Chip.

'Council's 'ere, spyin',' he called out. 'Wants to measure the sties. Give me a nasty feelin'. They might say pigs is not allowed.'

Chip measured the pigsties and convinced Miss Wilson that they were proper constructions, as approved by the council. She seemed genuinely delighted, not at all like the usual poker-faced council employee. They talked about pigs and vegetables, and Fred told her how the manure had benefited the allotments. Chip invited her to inspect his beans, and talked enthusiastically about the Dulwich Horticultural Show in two weeks' time. A pleasant hour was spent, and Miss Wilson left the two men happy with the feeling that the council would definitely approve of pigs on the allotments.

Chapter Twenty-Four

MR MOUNTSHAFT

But human happiness is too fragile to last. The following morning, the lady from the council's mother, Mrs Wilson, said to her daughter during breakfast: 'You're looking more cheerful this morning, dearie. I've been worried about you these last couple of weeks. Very quiet and thoughtful, you've been. It's nice to see you all smiling and cheerful again. Has anything been on your mind? Not Mr Mountshaft again, I hope?'

Miss Wilson was so relieved about the correctness of the size and structure of the pigsties that she told her mother everything. 'But you won't say anything to anyone, will you, Mum?'

'Of course not, dear, you can trust me.'

Mrs Wilson, of course, told her neighbour: 'But don't say a word, because she don't want it getting round.'

The neighbour told her cousin, who told a friend, who told the woman in the corner shop. Once a woman in a corner shop knows, you might as well publish the news in the *Daily Mirror*.

Forty-eight hours later, Mr Mountshaft entered the office.

'I hear there are pigs on the Mudchute allotments! Do you know anything about this, Miss Wilson? You were there a fortnight ago.'

Her mother's influence, and years of Sunday school during childhood, creating abhorrence of deceit, made her blush to the roots of her hair.

'Yes, Mr Mountshaft.'

'What?! You saw these animals a fortnight ago, and said nothing to me?'

'No, Mr Mountshaft,' she whispered.

'And why not, may I ask?'

Poor Miss Wilson – she couldn't reply, her voice had gone.

'This is out of order – a clear breach of council rules and regulations. Any irregularity occurring within council jurisdiction must be reported at once to a senior council employee. I will report this to the clerk responsible for Open Spaces and Leisure Activities, who has overall authority for the use of allotments. I have no doubt that he will take a very serious view of your conduct, Miss Wilson, and I must warn you that the matter could go as high as the town clerk.'

Poor Miss Wilson was trembling and looked on the verge of tears.

'In the meantime, take a letter, Miss Wilson. Address it to the man who rents the plot; inform him that pigs are not allowed on the Mudchute allotments, and that they must be removed by order, forthwith. Emphasise "by order". Bring the letter to me for signature.'

Mr Mountshaft turned to leave. Miss Wilson, the council doormat, had been suitably trodden on, and Mr Mountshaft felt satisfied.

But he was unaware of the inner steel of which his subordinate was made. He did not know that she had struggled through a poverty-stricken childhood; that she had lost three brothers and a father in the Second World War; that she had been an ambulance driver in the war and had faced much danger and witnessed much suffering; that she had educated herself through night school so that she could get a good job with a pension, and support her mother.

The steel came to the surface.

'Excuse me, Mr Mountshaft, but there is nothing in the

council regulations to say that pigs are not allowed on allotments.'

'What did you say?' Mr Mountshaft was startled. This was a new experience for him.

'There is nothing in the council regulations—'

'Yes, yes, I heard you. What do you mean?'

'I mean to point out what council regulations say.'

'I know perfectly well what the regulations say.'

Miss Wilson stood up. She needed to. This was the first time she had questioned her superior's authority, and she knew she had to be strong. Her voice was quiet, but very firm.

'I think you had better study the regulations before you send that letter, Mr Mountshaft. I have done so and can assure you that you are mistaken. Keeping pigs on allotments is not prohibited by the council. If you send that letter "by order" of the council, and you were in the wrong, the clerk responsible for Open Spaces and Leisure Activities would take a very serious view of your conduct, and the matter might be referred to the town clerk.'

Mr Mountshaft could not have been more astonished if one of the pigs in question had spoken to him. The council doormat had not only told him he was wrong, she had repeated his words and turned his threat upon himself. He swallowed hard and rubbed his finger around the inside of his collar.

'You had better give me a copy of the regulations relating to allotments, and I will study it.'

She handed him the documents in silence, and in silence he left the office.

Towards the evening, he returned. His voice was less arrogant and more respectful.

'I have studied the regulations, Miss Wilson, and I am bound to say you appear to be correct. Nonetheless, it all seems very irregular, and I shall request a meeting with the chief clerk in charge of Leisure Services early next week, when we will go into the matter more fully. In the meantime, I will see these pigs for myself.'

Accordingly, Mr Mountshaft took the bus to the Isle of Dogs after work. He looked so out of place on the allotments in his pin-striped suit, carrying a rolled umbrella on a hot summer's evening, that men working their plots knew at once that he was from the council. Nobby, the troublemaker, observed with quiet satisfaction that he walked straight to the corner plot. Fred was not there at the time, and Chip had not yet come off his shift in the docks, so Nobby reckoned he had the man from the council to himself. He let him survey the scene for a few minutes, take a few notes, and then he sidled up.

'Evenin', sir, fine evenin'. What's your verdic' abou' these 'ere pigs, then sir?' The question was put in a tone of voice that implied the answer was already known.

Mr Mountshaft eyed Nobby coolly. Rough-looking fellow, but probably no worse than the rest, he thought. He was not going to give anything away.

'Verdict? Well, er, let us see. What is your verdict and that of the other men on the allotments?'

'Lot o' grumblin', sir. We don't like to complain, we're not the sort to cause trouble, but since you're good enough to ask, sir, I can tell you there's a lo' o' blokes wha' don't like it. Not no way.'

He paused to see the effect of his words. Mr Mountshaft was still not going to show his hand. He wanted to hear for himself what the men had to say.

'Really?'

'Yes, really, sir. Lot o' grumblin'. These 'ere allotments are for growin' veggies, not for rearin' livestock. Where's it goin' to end? That's what the men says.'

'Indeed?'

'Yes, indeed, sir. I can tell you, sir, we're surprised the council ever gave permission for these pigs to come 'ere.'

'Are you?' said the man from the council.

'Yes. Don't seem right. But I suppose the council knows best, an' we jest 'ave to put up with the consequences. But I can tell you, sir, we're not 'appy abou' the situation.'

Nobby knew just when to stop. He touched his cap. 'Fine evenin', sir. Enjoy yer walk.' And he ambled off.

Mr Mountshaft had seen and heard enough. Unlike his female colleague, he was not in the least bit sentimental, and the sight of suckling piglets roused no maternal, or, to be more accurate, paternal instincts in him. He turned and left the allotments quickly. His roses in Wimbledon Common were more to his taste.

'There's been a man 'ere from the council, lookin' at yer pigs,' said Nobby to Fred, when he arrived.

'No?' said Fred in alarm.

'Straigh' up.' Nobby's face was impassive.

'What's 'e say?'

''Ow should I know? I never spoke to 'im.'

Chapter Twenty-Five

THE CHIEF CLERK

The clerk responsible for Dockland Redevelopment, Open Spaces and Leisure Activities had weighty matters to consider, and the use, or misuse, of allotments was not high on his list of priorities. When he received an internal memo from Mr Mountshaft informing him that pigs were being housed on the Mudchute allotments he was inclined to chuckle. Good luck to the fellow, he thought, and he threw the memo away. But when a second memo was handed to him, requesting a meeting, he felt obliged, reluctantly, to respond. Confound the man, pestering him when he had slum clearance on his mind.

Mr Mountshaft entered the large and imposing office of his superior. Senior council officials do rather well for themselves when it comes to sumptuous offices, and they can be very intimidating. Mr Mountshaft stood nervously before a huge mahogany desk, whilst the chief clerk continued writing and turning pages of a massive document. He continued in this way for a full two minutes, ignoring his visitor. It was a trick calculated to induce a feeling of inferiority, and poor Mr Mountshaft now felt both intimidated and inferior. Eventually the chief clerk looked up.

'We have a hundred and thirty acres of slums and derelict buildings to demolish, and two hundred thousand people to rehouse over the next three years. What a headache.' He closed the file and laid down his pen with a sigh. 'And what can I do for you?'

Mr Mountshaft shifted his feet uncomfortably.

'I'm sorry to trouble you, sir, so late in the day.'

'That is what I am here for,' said the chief clerk condescendingly and with a patient smile. 'The problems of my staff are my problems. Please go on.'

'It's about the Mudchute allotments.'

'Yes.'

'A man has rented an allotment and is keeping pigs on it.'

'And?'

'Well, that's it, sir. That's all.'

'Is this a problem, Mr Mountshaft?'

'It's highly irregular, sir.'

'Many things in life are irregular, Mr Mountshaft, but they do not amount to a problem. What do the regulations relating to the use of allotments have to say on pig breeding?'

'Nothing, sir.'

'Nothing?'

'No, sir.'

'Then there is no problem.'

'A section of land was designated by the council for the purpose of horticulture, sir, not for rearing livestock.'

'But do the regulations say the keeping of pigs is forbidden?'

'No, sir, they do not.'

'Then there is no problem – *Nisi interdictus est, licet.*'

'I beg your pardon, sir.'

'Oh, come now, you must know your Latin – *Nisi interdictus est, licet* or "That which is not forbidden is permitted".'

'But there are grumblings, sir. I have spoken to some of the men who rent the allotments and there is a great deal of discontent.' In point of fact, Mr Mountshaft had only spoken to one man, Nobby, and he only had Nobby's word for it that there were grumblings, but he saw no harm in exaggerating the level of discontent.

'Well, that puts a slightly different light on the matter – we can't have grumbling now, can we?'

'No, sir, we cannot.'

The chief clerk picked up his pen and gave thought to the matter.

'In that case I would like to meet the fellow who is keeping the pigs. Please instruct Miss Wilson to send the fellow a letter with an appointment to meet me. Also, I should like to see the relevant documents and archive material – please ask Miss Wilson to bring them to my office.'

The chief clerk reopened his file on slum clearance, to signal the end of the interview. Mr Mountshaft knew he was beaten and sidled out to give Miss Wilson her instructions.

Two days later, Fred received a letter on embossed vellum writing paper, and hadn't the faintest idea what it was all about. The only thing that was clear to him was that it involved pigs and allotments, and his immediate reaction was one of alarm and dismay – the council was going to get rid of them. In great agitation he brought the letter to Nonnatus House to consult his guide, philosopher and friend, who calmed his worst fears.

'Oh no,' said Sister Julienne, 'this is not about getting rid of your pigs. This is a summons from the chief clerk – he wants to meet you next week to discuss the matter, and if you have any sense, Fred, you will go.' Her firm voice and reassurance restored Fred's perky good humour.

On the day of the appointment he put on his only suit, an army demob relic, brushed his tooth, Brilliantined his hair, and looked real sharp. Pleased with his appearance, he made his way to the Poplar council offices, and with ten minutes to spare before the appointed hour he presented himself at the reception desk.

'Can I help you, sir?' asked a black-suited porter reproachfully.

'Well, I got an appointment wiv the chief clerk at ten o'clock. Look, it says so on this 'ere letter.'

He thrust the letter in the porter's face, rolled his fag across his lower lip and stared with his north-east eye at the porter, who took a step backwards in astonishment.

'It's about the allotments and pigs and manure and Chip's runner beans, and can pigs be kept on the allotment?'

Nonplussed, the porter could only murmur, 'Kindly follow me, sir.' He led Fred along a corridor with doors to left and right, up a staircase with a carved oaken balustrade, and along another corridor lined with more doors, each bearing a brass plate. Fred followed the immaculately dressed figure, grinning to himself and whistling through his tooth. The whistle was particularly penetrating and echoed around the corridors, causing the porter to wince.

Finally they stopped in front of a door with a small brass plate bearing the inscription 'Allotments'. They entered the office to find Miss Wilson sitting at her desk.

'This gentleman has an appointment with the chief clerk at ten o'clock. Will you kindly show him the way?' the porter said pompously.

Miss Wilson, who had been expecting Fred, rose from her chair with a smile and picked up her notebook and pen, as she was required to take minutes of the meeting. She led Fred, still whistling tunelessly, to an imposing door at the end of the corridor with a much larger brass plate bearing the inscription 'Dockland Redevelopment, Open Spaces and Leisure Activities'. She knocked on the door and while they waited she whispered, 'Good luck, hope it goes well.'

Fred, who was extremely confident, replied, 'Well, I reckons as 'ow we'll be all right. After all, I've got God on me side, can't go wrong – Sister Julienne and all the Sisters are praying for me.' When summoned, he gave her one of his saucy winks and together they entered the office, but not before he found a handy plant pot in which to stub out his cigarette!

Chapter Twenty-Six

THE MEETING

The chief clerk was sitting at his desk, dressed immaculately in pin-stripe suit, high collar, gold cufflinks and diamond tie pin. As they entered, some of Fred's confidence deserted him because, at a glance, he saw that he was no longer with an equal, but in the company of a 'gent'. Miss Wilson settled herself next to the desk ready to take the minutes. Fred remained standing.

'You wanted to see me, sir,' he said respectfully.

'Ah yes. Mr Wagstaff, I believe?'

'That's me, sir.'

'You live in Cubitt Town, on the Isle of Dogs, I believe?'

'Yessir.'

'And how long have you lived there?'

'All me life, sir. Born there, I was.'

'So you would describe yourself as an Islander?'

'Yessir. Me Mum and me Dad lived there an' all, sir.'

'Excellent. Most satisfactory.'

The chief clerk paused and glanced down at the documents on his desk, muttering something in Latin. Fred stood stiffly to attention, looking out of the window.

'And what is your occupation?'

'Well, I gets me livin' as best I can, sir.'

'You mean a bit of this and a bit of that?'

'Yessir. But legal, sir. Don't wan' no more brushes with the law, sir.'

'I see. Have you had brushes with the law, Mr Wagstaff?'

'Only the once, sir, when I made fireworks – but not no more.'

'Now your activities are strictly *manere dextrarus legis*, which means you like to keep on the right side of the law.'

'Yessir.'

Fred shifted his position sideways so that he could look at the chief clerk with his south-east eye.

'If you don't mind me sayin' so, sir, we 'ad a cove in the army, an officer like. Talked like you talk, foreign languages an' all.'

'Many people talk in foreign languages, Mr Wagstaff, but sadly Latin is dead.'

'Is that so, sir? Sorry to hear of anyone demisin', I am. I 'opes you don't feel the loss too sorely, sir?'

'All the time, Mr Wagstaff, all the time.' The chief clerk shook his head sadly and sighed.

'Now that's sad, real sad sir. If it's not an intrusion into your private sorrow, can I suggest you try gettin' out a bit more? Perks you up no end, it do, sir. When Mrs Wagstaff died, I was very low, bu' I perks meself up jest by getting out more.'

'You are a philosopher, Mr Wagstaff. An excellent piece of advice with endless ramifications. I feel better already. Have a cigarette.' He flicked open a gold cigarette case.

Fred took a cigarette and tucked it behind his ear. The chief clerk lit his, puffed a series of ephemeral smoke rings into the air, and watched them float upwards with evident satisfaction. He offered Fred his gold lighter.

'No, fank you, sir. I never smokes in the company of me betters. I'll enjoy it later.'

'As you wish. Well, now, we must return to the business in hand. I understand that you breed pigs?'

Fred hesitated. So this was it. They were on to him. He didn't know why, or what it was all about, but it meant trouble. Reluctantly he answered.

'Well, I got four pigs. Don't know as wha' they calls that breedin'.'

'Only four?'

'Yessir. Blossom, Blackberry, Bluebell an' Chrystaline.'

'They sound like pets.'

'Yessir, 'specially Blossom. She's the oldest. I've 'ad 'er longest, see? Lovely nature, she's got, lovely nature. Real 'uman, she is.'

'And where do you keep them?'

This was the question Fred has been dreading. He sighed deeply. The end was in sight.

'On the allotments, sir.' His voice was very low.

'The allotments?'

'Yessir.'

The chief clerk shuffled some papers. For the first time, Fred noticed a pile of yellow-looking parchments on the desk, and some maps. He was obliged to look sideways in order to see them out of his south-west eye. He jerked stiffly to attention again.

'And did you ask the council's permission to take your pigs to the allotments?'

There was a long pause.

'Did you?'

'No, sir.'

'You just assumed the right to take them to the allotments?'

'Yessir. Reckons as 'ow I did, sir.'

The chief clerk slapped both hands down on the desk, scattering the yellow parchments. 'Splendid, splendid! *Noli quarere, carpe diem.*'

'Wassat, sir?'

'It means "Don't ask, seize the opportunity", or perhaps more colloquially, "Don't ask, just take".'

'Well, I suppose I did, sir. No one said as what I couldn't, like.'

'Exactly! *Nisi interdictus est, licet.* Which means "That which is not forbidden is permitted".'

'Well, that's real nice to know,' Fred said, sucking his tooth thoughtfully. 'Me mates'll be right glad to 'ear that one, comin' from a gent like you, sir.'

'I have just a few more questions, Mr Wagstaff, which I hope you can answer.'

'I'll do me best, sir.'

'What do you do with your pigs?'

'Well, the piglets go to market, when they're big enough, like, an' the manure goes to the other blokes on the allotments.'

'So your fellow allotment holders benefit from the keeping of pigs, in that they use the manure?'

'Reckons as 'ow they do, sir.'

Again the chief clerk slapped the desk.

'*Salus populi suprema est lex*!' he cried triumphantly.

'Wassat, sir?'

'It means "The good of the people is the first law".'

'Oh yeah, sounds all right to me.'

'Indeed, Mr Wagstaff, it is very all right. "The greatest good for the greatest number" – John Stuart Mill, eighteen six to eighteen seventy-three, philosopher and economist. Your pigs are of benefit to the production of edible comestibles from the manure they produce.'

'Wassat, sir?'

'The manure helps the vegetables grow.'

'Yessir.'

'By common consent your fellow allotment holders approve the keeping of pigs?'

'Yes, sir, by an' large, wiv one or two exceptions, but most of them approve of 'em on the allotments.' Fred chose not to mention Nobby and his small band of malcontents, and saw no harm in exaggerating the level of content.

'Allotments are a reasonable place for the keeping of pigs?'

'Well, yessir. Enough space, but not on top o' you, like.'

'Splendid! Splendid! Mr Wagstaff, I am confident in saying that you have every right to keep your pigs on the allotments, and may continue doing so. If anyone tells you to the contrary, take no notice. The council may assume bureaucratic rights, but your rights as an Islander are of greater antiquity and established as a local custom. *Nisi interdictus est, licet.* That which is not forbidden is permitted, Mr Wagstaff. *Jus plebis.* Which means "The rights of the People", Mr Wagstaff.'

'That's a relief, sir, I don't mind tellin' yer. Reckoned as 'ow you was goin' to tell me to get rid o' me pigs. Break me 'eart, it would've done. It's been a real pleasure meetin' you, sir. A gent like you doesn't pop up every day. Real pleasure.'

They shook hands and Fred departed, whistling all the way down the stairs, through the corridors and out through the doors. The penetrating sound of his whistling could be heard long after the little figure was well out of sight.

The chief clerk sighed and turned his attention back to the problems of clearing a hundred and thirty acres of slum buildings, and of two hundred thousand people to rehouse over the next three years.

Miss Wilson could quite easily have given the chief clerk a great big hug, so pleased was she with the outcome of the meeting, but she restrained herself; it was more than her position was worth to be hugging the chief clerk! Instead she closed her notebook, replaced the lid of her pen and went in search of Mr Mountshaft to break the news.

Chapter Twenty-Seven

WORD SPREADS

Miss Wilson was quietly thrilled at the outcome of the meeting, and couldn't wait to see the look on Mr Mountshaft's face when she broke the news. Needless to say, Mr Mountshaft was furious, and stormed and raged about his office, kicking over the wastepaper bin in the process, scattering its contents all over the place. Miss Wilson couldn't help but chuckle at his reaction, and the look on his face was a picture.

'I can't see what there is to laugh at,' snapped Mr Mountshaft.

'No, sir. Just thoughts. Nothing to do with work, sir.'

Miss Wilson had to turn away to hide her amusement, and Mr Mountshaft glared suspiciously at her back. Had that impudent woman got something to do with the unexpected turn of events? She was a dark horse. Did she know more than she was letting on? He wouldn't be surprised. He would have to watch out for her.

After work, Miss Wilson did not go straight home. Instead, she took a stroll down to the Isle of Dogs. The sun was warm and bright, having lost its midday heat. The streets were hot and smoky, but once she reached the allotments the air became clear and fresh.

The allotments looked beautiful in the evening light. They were lush and green and sweet-smelling, and a lot of men were working, making last-minute improvements to their produce for the Dulwich Horticultural Show the following

Saturday. Sparrows were hopping around everywhere, squabbling and twittering. The lady from the council walked directly to the pigsties, where Fred was mucking out. He turned as she approached. His curious face, with his eyes that looked in two directions, his one yellow tooth, a fag end drooping from the corner of his mouth, and his crooked grin reminded her of an amiable gargoyle on the high cornices of a cathedral, the sort that can be seen only through binoculars.

She went straight up to him and congratulated him on the news, emphasising that it had been proved beyond doubt that he had the right to keep his pigs on the allotments, and that he was supported by the law.

Fred vaulted over the wall of the sty, put two grubby, smelly hands on her shoulders and kissed her, with the words, 'You darlin'! Yer an angel!'

Miss Wilson, who had not been kissed spontaneously in that way since a spotty youth had kissed her on the cheek during a Sunday school outing, blushed to the roots of her hair.

Fred, who had been keeping the news to himself up until that point, could contain himself no longer. He shouted, 'Oy, Chip, come 'ere. Lady from the council's go' some news. Come over 'ere.'

Several men heard the shout, and followed Chip over to the pigsties to hear the news. Fred, proud and excited, told them. 'We won! We can keep the pigs, an' it's go' the law behind it, an' all, ain't it, miss?'

Still blushing, Miss Wilson confirmed that it had.

There was a whoop of excitement, and the men lifted Fred shoulder-high and carried him down the little paths, all around the allotments and back again. By the time they got back, word had spread and there was not one allotment holder that had not heard the news.

Miss Wilson did not join them. She stood by the pigsty and watched the scene with quiet satisfaction, aware that she had been instrumental in keeping the pigs in their home. Mr Mountshaft would have had them out two weeks ago, and no one would have said a word about ancient rights. She let out a sigh of satisfaction and turned to gaze one last time at the pigs. Perhaps she ought to go. Her mother would be expecting her in the little terraced house they shared in Camden. Whilst the men were still cheering Fred, she slipped quietly away.

The triumphal procession carrying Fred around the allotments confirmed his popularity. The Dulwich Horticultural Show was in everyone's thoughts, and the glories of prize-winning vegetables were all around them. Fred's contribution, or rather his pigs' contribution, was indisputable and his supporters swelled in number, including some of Nobby's previous malcontents, who had switched allegiance. They were jubilant and, in marked contrast to the usual quiet, stolid temperament of dedicated allotment diggers, were almost rowdy.

One observer, however, did not join the procession. Nobby Clark was seething with suppressed fury. He didn't like noise, couldn't get on with shouting and laughing, and didn't go in for cheering. His own band of supporters was shrinking, and he ground his teeth in impotent rage when he heard 'For He's a Jolly Good Fellow' being sung. He picked up a stone to hurl it at the pigs. He turned and took aim; but in that instant his arm dropped and the stone fell from his hand. He stared long and hard at the pigsties, and slowly a twisted smile crept over his sour features.

During the dark and silent hours of night between Thursday sunset and Friday sunrise, Nobby Clark slipped out of his little terraced house, made his way to the allotments, to the pigsties, opened the gates, and returned to his bed.

Chapter Twenty-Eight

FRED'S DOWNFALL

The cockerel was first to greet the dawn with his shrill cry, ducks opened their eyes and quacked; sparrows chirped a reedy sound, but they quickly found their voices and a chorus of birdsong filled the air. Rustling was heard in the bushes, and small creatures started about their business for the day.

Four sows, fifteen mature piglets and fourteen newborn piglets awoke, grunting and snuffling and lumbering about their sties. In the darkness they could not see that the gates were open, but as the sun rose they became aware of the opening and peered out. They stepped tentatively out into the new and vast world beyond the walls of their sties, uncertain of what to do or where to go. One mature piglet, bolder than the rest, ventured about ten yards down a path and found a row of carrots. Soon he was digging and eating them up happily. His piglet brothers and sisters followed him and, in no time, not only the carrots, but the turnips, swedes and parsnips, the pride and joy of their owner's heart, had all been devoured. Prize onions, due to be pulled the next day for the show, were rooted up and left scattered around.

Chrystaline, the milking sow, followed by her fourteen suckling piglets, walked heavily on her dainty trotters across five or six plots, her sharp blades digging deep into the soft earth at every step. Several beds of lettuces, spring onions, trailing cucumbers and French beans were demolished. She reached Plot 58, and the demands of her squealing brood forced her to lie down suddenly and heavily into a bed of marrow plants. The piglets soon attached themselves to her teats and the sow, smelling a very large marrow just where she was lying, chewed it contentedly.

Blossom and Blackberry, who was heavily pregnant, came across a trellis of fine runner beans, where they ate all the lower beans. Then Blossom became aware of beans growing higher up; she stretched her neck to get at them, and then raised herself on her hind legs, resting her front trotters against the verdant green leafage. The trellis collapsed. The pigs ate all the beans they wanted, and then continued foraging. Bluebell found a potato plot and, within fifteen minutes, had dug up the lot, eating some and leaving the rest to lie.

Meanwhile, the fifteen mature piglets, with full stomachs and the exuberance of youth, were playing on plots near to the river. Piglets will gambol and play like lambs if they get the chance, and they can run surprisingly fast. They were running and jumping and chasing each other, tearing through beds of prime cabbages, Brussels sprouts, leeks and curly kale. They dug deep just for the fun of it, showering the earth into piles behind them, like a dog burying a bone. They ripped at peas, tearing and shaking them, but the tomatoes fared worst. As everyone knows, it is hard to grow tomatoes in these northern climes, but that year, with continuous sunshine, and tender loving care, they were outstandingly fine, turning from green to delicate orange. The piglets, attracted by the colour, made a dive for them. And that was the end of the tomatoes.

At 6 a.m. on that fateful Friday, two men dropped by the allotments on their way to work. Number 58 wanted to check his marrows, which he planned to cut on Saturday morning, the day of the Dulwich Horticultural Show. His companion was looking across the river as they strolled along.

'Fine morning, ain't it?'

'Lovely. None better.'

'D'ya see that boat?'

He heard a shriek.

'What the bloody hell!'

'What?'

'Look! A bloody pig's got loose.'

'Where?'

'In me marrers.'

Number 58 was running. He picked up a stone and hurled it at Chrystaline. She looked up and raised herself on her haunches in surprise. She was accustomed to tender endearments from Fred, and admiration from human beings generally. She could not conceive that one of the species could throw stones. The man picked up another, and threw it with force. It struck her between the eyes, and she leaped up with a shriek and made off at a gallop across the allotments. The piglets, who had been peacefully sleeping, scattered, squealing and running around in circles, utterly destroying those of the marrow plants that so far had escaped damage.

Number 58 howled with as much anguish as the injured pig. He walked amongst his destroyed plants, picking up one or two in despair. He turned his beautiful marrow, the one that was a prize winner, and saw that a quarter of it had been chewed away. He sat on the ground and wept.

His companion looked around at the devastation. He was not a plot owner, nor a fanatic, but he could see that the damage was extensive.

'Good Gawd! They're everywhere. Look.'

He pointed to the fifteen mature piglets gambolling in the sweetcorn.

'Someone had better tell Fred.'

He dashed off to Fred's terraced house and banged on the door, but there was no reply. He threw a pebble at the upstairs window and shouted.

'You best get up mate, yer pigs 'as got loose.'

Fred came to the window.

'Wha' choo say?'

'Yer pigs is everywhere. Got loose some'ow.'

'Oh my good Gawd!' swore Fred, struggling into his trousers, but taking care with his zip, having had a nasty experience with one when he was a young man.

It had been a hot night, and the windows were open all down the street. Seconds later, men were at the windows shouting the news to one another. Front doors were banging as they raced out of little houses and down the narrow streets. Someone banged on Chip's door as he passed.

'Pigs loose on the allotments. It's right bloody carnage.'

Within minutes everyone knew the story, and by 6.15 a.m. around thirty men were on the allotments, surveying the devastation of their hopes and dreams with disbelief, despair, or blind rage.

'Round 'em up!' someone shouted.

The men gave chase, which created panic amongst the pigs. They charged around the place, dodging and weaving from their pursuers, thereby destroying what had been left undamaged. Blossom, Blackberry and Bluebell were the first captured, because they were slowest, but the mature piglets were another matter. They were sixteen weeks old, fast, agile and resourceful.

Two of them, chased by three men, ran at high speed into the side of a chicken coop and demolished it, sending chickens and feathers flying everywhere. Their distraught owner rushed around trying to catch them, but in vain. Of the original dozen, only two hens were ever caught. The others vanished without trace.

A couple of men thought they could round up the baby piglets, which were clustered together squealing pathetically. They were picking them up when Chrystaline saw what was going on. With the instincts of a mother and a roar more like a bull than a pig, she charged. She hit one man full frontal and he fell, winded and wounded. Then she turned on the other man. Seeing the villainous gleam in her eyes, he dropped the piglets and ran, chased by the pig. His heavy feet destroyed a bed of succulent strawberries, and another of ripening melons. He didn't feel safe until he was at least three streets away.

One's heart must bleed for poor Fred. His concern was all for his beloved pigs. He wasn't interested in vegetables, and could not share the anguish of the men.

Chrystaline was eventually caught and returned to the sty, and the baby piglets followed their mother. But of the original fifteen mature piglets, only four were ever caught. Three leaped into the Thames and swam off at a fair rate of knots towards Tower Bridge (it is commonly thought that pigs cannot swim, but this is an error). The rest found their way out of the allotment gates and charged down West Ferry Road, like a band of headstrong teenagers. Four made it as far as the docks and were later found sleeping peacefully on the wharf. The remaining eight reached the East India Dock Road, which is a major arterial road, and ten policemen and several nippy lads attempted to catch them. The traffic was held up for more than an hour and they were never seen again.

By eight o'clock, some sort of peace was restored. The four sows and all the newborn piglets were back in their sties and the gates firmly shut. Fred was with them, tending to the wound between Chrystaline's eyes, thankful only that most of them were back. The men, who had work to get to, were leaving the allotment. They made a point of passing the sties, shaking their fists and cursing poor Fred. For his part, Fred could not understand their anger.

When Chip came up to him and muttered through clenched teeth, 'This is the end, this is,' Fred's innocent reply was:

'You can grow some more.'

'Not in time for the Dulwich show tomorrow, you fool.'

Chapter Twenty-Nine

ALL IS NOT LOST

The men who were left, who didn't have work to get to, decided something must be done. An angry crowd stormed the council rooms demanding in language that cannot be repeated that the allotments be cleared of pigs. Fred, fearful he might be beaten up if he followed them, crept home. He trembled and kept indoors behind drawn curtains.

The following morning brought a letter from the council, requiring him to remove his pigs from the allotments and giving him three working days in which to do so.

On Sunday morning, early, when he knew that his neighbours would be having a lie-in, Fred fearfully left his house, and with head down and collar turned up he made his way stealthily to the convent. We were surprised to see him. His duties as boiler man did not include Sundays. The Sisters were in chapel. He let himself in the back door, for which he had a key, and entered the kitchen where we girls were having breakfast.

'What ho! This is an unexpected pleasure,' cried Chummy cheerfully.

Fred did not answer, but looked fearfully all around as though expecting an allotment holder with a fist of steel to leap out at him.

'Where's Sister Julienne?' he whispered hoarsely.

'She's in chapel, old bean.'

'Oh yes, o'course. I'll wait. Shall I wait 'ere? Or will I sit in the coal shed?' he asked meekly.

His voice and his whole aspect were so unusual that we immediately felt alarmed.

Cynthia spoke. 'Wait here, of course. You can't go and sit in the coal shed. Sit here with us and have a cup of tea.' She poured one and added three sugars. 'What's the matter, Fred?' she asked gently as she handed him the mug. He tried to speak but only a croaking whisper came out of his dry lips, no words.

'Drink your tea, Fred. Don't try to talk if you don't want to.' Cynthia was always intuitive and kind.

We sat eating our breakfast with Fred sitting apart on a chair by the boiler, sipping his tea. His head was bent, and he just stared at the tiled floor. Every so often we heard a sniff, followed by a prolonged and noisy nose blowing.

Voices were heard in the corridor, and four Sisters entered the kitchen. The tragic figure of Fred caught their attention. Sister Julienne came over to him and enquired what had happened.

'It's me pigs,' was all he could say, in a subdued whisper, as he pulled a letter from his pocket and handed it to her. She read it in silence.

'This is an order from the council, telling you to remove the pigs within three days. Do you know why this has happened, Fred?'

In hoarse and faltering tones, punctuated by long pauses and choking sounds, he told us. No one laughed. It would have been too cruel to laugh at the little man. His distress was making him ill. Sister Julienne's face looked really angry when he had finished.

'This sounds like a deliberate act of mischief, or malice. You might have left one gate insecure, but not all four. Someone opened all the gates in the night on purpose to harm you, Fred. It's monstrous. Have you any idea who might have done it?'

'I've a fair idea,' mumbled Fred as he shook his head and blew his nose again.

'And I don't suppose the villain will ever be caught,' Sister continued, 'and even if he was, I doubt if any magistrate could bring a charge against him. I think this has got something to do with the Dulwich Horticultural Show. There is no end to what jealousy between rival competitors will lead to. They called it "nobbling" or "spiking" a man's chances of winning when I was a child, and it was always nasty.'

She read the letter again, and gave it back to Fred.

'Well, this is an order; there is nothing you can do about it. I think you had better ask the breeder in Essex if he will take them. Come into my office to make the phone call.' She paused and looked thoughtful. 'You know, Fred, it's suddenly struck me. You don't need to get rid of all your pigs. Why not keep Blossom in your backyard, just as you did before. You will enjoy her company all the more when there are just the two of you.'

Fred perked up for the first time that morning, and his mouth worked into a twisted grin. He may have been despondent, crushed by the blow from the council, but he was also a Cockney, born and bred into wrestling with a fate that seemed determined to get him. He had spent half his life rising like a cross-eyed phoenix from the ashes of disaster, and withal he was an incurable optimist. He jumped up.

'You've gottit, Sister. Blossom, me beauty. Why didn' I fink of it? I don't need four pigs – lot o' muckin' out an' feedin' in the winter. Just me and Blossom, that's the answer.'

If he had had the nerve, I think he would have kissed her – but it takes an awful lot of nerve for a man to kiss a nun!

The following day, the long-suffering Essex farmer loaded Fred's pigs on to his truck. He drove first to Fred's house and unloaded Blossom. She seemed to know where she was and needed no coaxing to go down the narrow passage, around the corner, and into the yard. With a grunt of satisfaction, she looked at her old sty and walked straight to it, snorting contentedly. Fred had filled a trough of bran, and she dipped her snout in and began eating noisily. Fred scratched her back, and she lifted her head and looked at him with a gleam in her small, bright eyes.

'Welcome home, ole lady,' said Fred. And the pig chortled, as only pigs can.

Chapter Thirty

THE LADY IN ESSEX

Time passes, and London was changing fast in the decade after the Second World War. The confidence and light-hearted freedom of those post-war years could not last for ever. The East End of London had to be rebuilt, and bureaucracy, planning permission and restrictions came with it. Inevitably, Fred's contentment with Blossom in his backyard came to the attention of the Health and Hygiene boys, and she had to go – a danger to public health, they said.

Fred was distraught at the thought of losing his beloved Blossom and he poured out his sorrows to anyone who would listen. Once again, Sister Julienne came up with a solution – why not ask the farmer from Essex if he would have her? Fred could visit as often as he liked.

Arrangements were made and the farmer from Essex arrived with his truck to pick up Blossom – he very much hoped it would be the last time he ever had to make this particular journey. Fred visited often and we all wondered at his devotion. But old age catches up with us all, including pigs, and Blossom was getting to be an old lady. When she died, Fred's visits continued, however, and we knew there must be more to it than a pig.

When he started smartening himself up, we girls looked at each other knowingly. When he bought a new suit, some white shirts, several rather garish ties and some suede shoes, we knew that something was up. When he had his single yellowing tooth removed, and dentures fitted, we knew he was serious.

The false teeth were quite startling. To begin with, there seemed to be so many of them – far more than the usual complement of teeth given to us by nature, and their pearly whiteness was dazzling. In the mouth of a young person they would not look out of place, but in the mouth of a man in his late fifties, with his weather-beaten skin and decidedly odd appearance, they looked singularly out of place. Not that Fred was aware of this – he was hugely pleased and flashed his smile at everyone.

Eating had been a problem, he confided, but he reckoned he could get round that one with a bit of practice. His speech was also affected – having spent most of his life with only one tooth, his speech had adapted, but his new teeth presented him with a challenge. He'd have to get round that one with a bit of practice as well. His toothbrush, which had served him well since before the war, was finally replaced.

Unfortunately the teeth weren't a perfect fit. Every so often they would slip, either when he was smiling or talking, which he did often, and the effect was comical to say the very least. It was hard not to laugh at him, but that would have hurt his pride, so we girls had to suppress our giggles and titters.

'There's this bit wot rubs at the back,' he complained. He would have to go back to the dentist and get it sorted.

'Marvellous this new NHS,' he declared, 'brand-new choppers and nothing to pay, just marvellous! But still, there shouldn't be a bit wot rubs, should there? Can't have dodgy choppers, can I?'

We all agreed it was marvellous, but, no, you can't have dodgy choppers, and so off he went to the dentist to have the bit that was rubbing rubbed off.

We debated how we could discreetly enquire into the purpose of this transformation. It would not be easy, but we were just about dying with curiosity. One Friday, Fred turned up at the convent in a new suit, new shirt with matching tie, new trilby, new shoes and his flashing teeth.

'Will yer gives Sister Julienne a message for me? Will yer tells 'er I'll not be in over the weekend as I'm on me way to Essex?'

Trixie could contain her curiosity no longer, and blurted out, 'Oh, come on Fred, out with it: who is she?'

He rubbed his nose artfully and replied, 'Ask no questions an' I'll tell yer no lies.'

Try as we might we could draw no further clues from him.

But Fred did tell us when he got back – he could keep no secrets, and he could never stop talking either. To keep a good story to himself would have been out of character.

It was Monday morning, and we all were sitting round the big kitchen table having breakfast, whilst Fred, in his old shirt and overalls, was raking out the stove.

Trixie fired the first shot.

'Come on, Fred, you owe us an explanation. Who is the lady and what's she like?'

Fred needed no nudging.

'Well, she's a widow-lady, respectable like. Lost 'er 'usband in the war. Lives wiv 'er dad at The Crafty Fox.'

'The Crafty Fox?'

'Like I said, The Crafty Fox. It's a pub in Matching Tye in Essex. 'Er dad's the landlord an' all.'

'Don't be ridiculous, Fred, there's no such place as Matching Tie. You went to Essex wearing one. There can't be a place named after one!' The play on words was completely lost on Fred and he continued poking at the stove.

'I'm telling yer, Matching Tye. It's a village in Essex, near where the farm was where Blossom was kept. Well, she's the barmaid o' course an' very nice she is too. Now, stop bovering me wiv yer silly questions, I've got raking to do.'

'Sorry, Fred, but how long have you known her?'

'Reckons about six months, all told.'

'This is all very interesting. You're a sly one, Fred.'

Fred accepted the compliment graciously.

This was too good to be true. The Crafty Fox! Trixie had just accused Fred of being something similar. And Matching Tie? It just couldn't be possible – Fred must be having us on. We girls looked at one another and resolved to investigate further.

'Well, she's a nice bit o' stuff, proper lady, like, an' I don't 'ang about when I sees a nice bit o' stuff. We're walking out, you understand, walking out.'

We had none of us envisaged Fred as a Casanova amongst women, but maybe we felt the prejudice of youth.

'Interesting. And what do you do when you're not walking out?'

Trixie could be very blunt.

Fred was indignant. 'What d'ya finks we do? When we're not walking out, she's serving the customers in the bar, an' I'm sitting at the bar chatting up the customers and singin' a few o' me songs.' Fred's busking days were long since gone, but he still liked to think of himself as a bit of a singer.

'Sounds like a good arrangement.'

''Tis an' all, very nice, very comfortable. They tells me business has really picked up, can't fink why.'

Can't think why? We girls could think why – a too-good-to-be-true Cockney in their midst, singing songs. No wonder business had picked up! But Fred was totally unaware of his peculiar charms, and would say nothing more. He finished his raking and clattered out with his bucket of ash.

Fred's pattern of weekend visits to Essex continued, and we girls expected to hear news of wedding bells, but no. One day Trixie said impulsively: 'Now Fred, let's have it: when are you going to pop the question?' To which Fred replied with a good-humoured flash of his teeth, 'I'm tellin' yer, there'll be no popping of questions, no way. No' now, no' never. We're walkin' out, see, walkin' out.'

Time passes and London continued to change with ever-increasing rapidity. One by one the docks closed, and the dockers were made redundant. Slum clearance, which had begun in the 1950s, stepped up a pace in the 1960s, and many people were rehoused in the New Towns, tearing apart the extended family that had provided the unity and strength of the East Enders for generations.

The changes affected the Sisters' practice significantly, particularly the NHS and the fashion for having babies in hospital. The advent of the Pill in 1964 reduced the birth rate from around one hundred per month to around four. They closed their midwifery and nursing practice, but continued working, serving the varied and ever-changing needs of the local community.

For nearly one hundred years, the Sisters had served God and the people of Poplar. For nearly sixty of those years, Fred had faithfully served the Sisters. When asked about the lady in Essex, he simply replied: 'The Sisters need me, can't let them down, now, can I? Reckons as 'ow I'll stay 'ere until they don't need me no more.'

In 1978, Nonnatus House was closed – the Sisters' work was done, and with it Fred's work was done. The Sisters moved to the Mother House, to await God's next calling. Fred, approaching his eighties, moved to Matching Tye in Essex to be with his widow-lady. As far as anyone knows, they continued walking out for the rest of their days.

ACKNOWLEDGEMENTS

There are inevitably a great many people to thank, both past and present.

To begin with, I must thank Merton Books for first bringing *Call the Midwife* to public attention; Eugenie Furness and Kirsty Dunseath for spotting its potential and bringing it to a much wider audience and Neal Street Productions for bringing it to the widest possible audience.

This book was really just an idea I had during lockdown. Therefore special thanks must go to my cousin Sarah for encouraging me to pursue that idea, and seeing where it would go. I have to thank Maddy Price and all the team at Orion Publishing for their enthusiasm when I first floated the idea, and for turning it into a reality.

I would like to thank Chris Shelley for his photographic expertise and Sarah Ford for her computer know-how and technical back-up. Also, thank you to Maria Honeycombe for reading the first draft of my foreword.

My sister Juliette and my daughters Lydia and Eleanor deserve extra-special thanks for their ongoing support and encouragement.

Above all, I would like to thank my parents; each of them an inspiration in their own way. I like to think of them smiling down on us, holding hands and feeling proud.

PICTURE CREDITS

A true story of the East End in the 1950s

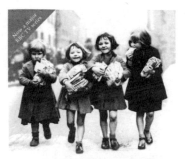

a true story of the east end
in the 1950s

Call the Midwife

JENNIFER WORTH

Jennifer Worth came from a sheltered background when she became a midwife in the Docklands in the 1950s. The conditions in which many women gave birth just half a century ago were horrifying, not only because of their grimly impoverished surroundings, but also because of what they were expected to endure. But while Jennifer witnessed brutality and tragedy, she also met with amazing kindness and understanding, tempered by a great deal of Cockney humour. She also earned the confidences of some whose lives were truly stranger, more poignant and more terrifying than could ever be recounted in fiction.

Funny, disturbing and incredibly moving, Jennifer's stories bring to life the colourful world of the East End in the 1950s.

'Full of fascinating social history'
New Statesman

**A fascinating slice of East End life, from the
no.1 bestselling author of *Call the Midwife***

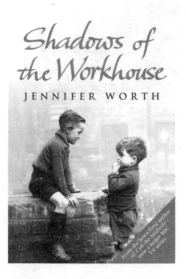

In this follow-up to *Call the Midwife*, Jennifer Worth, a midwife
working in the docklands area of east London in the 1950s, tells
more stories about the people she encountered.

There's Jane, who cleaned and generally helped out at Nonnatus
House – she was taken to the workhouse as a baby and was allegedly
the illegitimate daughter of an aristocrat. Peggy and Frank's parents
both died within 6 months of each other and the children were left
destitute. At the time, there was no other option for them but the
workhouse. The Reverend Thornton-Appleby-Thorton, a missionary in Africa, visits the Nonnatus nuns and Sister Julienne acts as
matchmaker. And Sister Monica Joan, the eccentric 90-year-old nun,
is accused of shoplifting some small items from the local market.

These stories give a fascinating insight into the resilience and
spirit that enabled ordinary people to overcome their difficulties.

'Worth's portrait is subtle, skilfully describing a sense of community that no longer exists'
Financial Times

The third and final book in the bestselling
Call the Midwife series

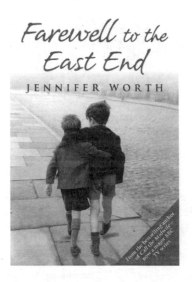

This final book in Jennifer Worth's memories of her time as a midwife in London's East End brings her story full circle. As always there are heartbreaking stories, as well as plenty of humour and warmth.

We discover what happens with the gauche debutant Chummy and her equally gauche policeman; will Sister Monica Joan continue her life of crime? Will Sister Evangelina ever crack a smile? And what of Jennifer herself? The book not only details the final years of the tenements but also of Jennifer's journey as she moves on from the close community of nuns she has been working with, and her life takes a new path.

'Worth is a vivid writer with a talent for the sting in the tail
. . . a highly readable book'
Evening Standard

What makes a good death?

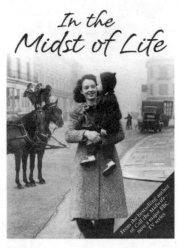

JENNIFER WORTH

In the Midst of Life

From the bestselling author of *Call the Midwife* — now a major BBC TV series

Jennifer Worth's bestselling memoirs of her time as a midwife have inspired and moved readers of all ages. Now, in *In the Midst of Life* she documents her experiences as a nurse and ward sister, treating patients who were nearing the end of their lives. Interspersed with these stories from Jennifer's post-midwife career are the histories of her patients, from the family divided by a decision nobody could bear to make, to the mother who comes to her son's adopted country and joins his family without being able to speak a word of English.

In the Midst of Life gives moving insights not just into Jennifer's life and career, but also of a period of time which seems very different to today's, fast-paced world.

'Worth is indeed a natural storyteller . . . gripping, moving and convincing from beginning to end . . . a powerful evocation of a long-gone world'
Literary Review

A lovely collection of letters to Jennifer Worth, diary entries, photos and an introduction by Miranda Hart

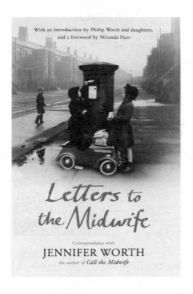

Letters to the Midwife is a wonderful collection of correspondence received by Jennifer Worth, offering a fascinating glimpse into a long-lost world and filled with all sorts of heart-warming gems. There are stories from other midwives, lorry drivers, even a seamstress, all with tales to tell.

Containing previously unpublished material describing her time spent in Paris and some journal entries, this is also a portrait of Jennifer herself, complete with a moving introduction by her family about the woman they knew and loved.

'Touching and irreverent . . . [a] testament to the huge affection she inspired – and to how unerringly accurate her portrayal of a fast-vanishing world was'
Mail on Sunday